zen

and the art of
DIABETES
MAINTENANCE

a
spiritual
toolkit
for a
better life

CHARLES CREEKMORE

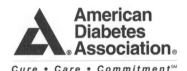

American
Diabetes
Association®

Cure • Care • Commitment℠

Director, Book Publishing, John Fedor; *Associate Director, Consumer Books,* Sherrye Landrum; *Editor,* Abe Ogden; *Production Manager,* Peggy M. Rote; *Composition,* Circle Graphics; *Cover Design,* Design Literate, Inc.; *Printer,* Transcontinental Printing

Printed in Canada
1 3 5 7 9 10 8 6 4 2

The suggestions and information contained in this publication are generally consistent with the *Clinical Practice Recommendations* and other policies of the American Diabetes Association, but they do not represent the policy or position of the Association or any of its boards or committees. Reasonable steps have been taken to ensure the accuracy of the information presented. However, the American Diabetes Association cannot ensure the safety or efficacy of any product or service described in this publication. Individuals are advised to consult a physician or other appropriate health care professional before undertaking any diet or exercise program or taking any medication referred to in this publication. Professionals must use and apply their own professional judgment, experience, and training and should not rely solely on the information contained in this publication before prescribing any diet, exercise, or medication. The American Diabetes Association—its officers, directors, employees, volunteers, and members—assumes no responsibility or liability for personal or other injury, loss, or damage that may result from the suggestions or information in this publication.

♾ The paper in this publication meets the requirements of the ANSI Standard Z39.48-1992 (permanence of paper).

ADA titles may be purchased for business or promotional use or for special sales. For information, please write to Lee Romano Sequeira, Special Sales & Promotions, at the address below.

American Diabetes Association
1701 North Beauregard Street
Alexandria, Virginia 22311

Library of Congress Cataloging-in-Publication Data
Creekmore, Charles, 1945-
  Zen and the art of diabetes maintenance / Charles Creekmore.
    p. cm.
  Includes index.
  ISBN 1-58040-120-1 (pbk. :alk. paper)
    1. Diabetes—Popular works. 2. Diabetes—Psychological aspects. 3. Spiritual life. I. Title

RC660.4 .C74 2002
616.4'62'0019—dc21

2002018221

Dedicated to
Martha Lee Michalek,
the keeper of my faith

Contents

Acknowledgments

I would like to express my sincere thanks to the many people who, both knowingly and unknowingly, helped me conceptualize, research, and write this book.

First of all, let me acknowledge several authors, editors, and wise people whose spiritual ideas I have studied and quoted: Lama Surya Das, Thomas Moore, His Holiness the Dalai Lama, Dr. Howard Cutler, Dr. Deepak Chopra, Professor Philip Zaleski, Dr. Herbert Benson, Steve Hagen, Professor Phyllis D. Rose, Dr. Jon Kabat-Zinn, and Bill Moyers.

I owe another debt of gratitude to a number of medical professionals who have assisted in this writing project: Dr. Harold G. Koenig, Dr. David B. Larson,

Craig M. Broadhurst, Paula S. Yutzy, Dr. Valerie Yancey, and Dr. Warren Morgan.

I also appreciate the invaluable help of eight people with diabetes who contributed their experiences and their wisdom to my book: Jewett Pattee, Reverend Edward Schroeder, Michael Jessup, Rod Frantz, Vicki Gaubeca, Michael Raymond, Joe Clifford, and Jim Collins.

In addition, I'd like to thank the loyal friends who have supported me in this and other writing projects over the years: Terry Allen, Ernie Urvater, Robert Abel, Tom Fix, Richard Farrell, Rachel Morton, Steve Long, Liz Pols, Al Hall, Jody Pritchard, Bob Clark, Sue and Tom Brando, Sharon Scott Hawkins, Keith McCormick, Alexey Veraksa, Jay Harrington, Jo Burns, Sister Frances Randall, and Allen Blair.

Many thanks also go to my family for decades of long-term nurturing: my mother Mary Lee Koltz, my brother Tony Koltz, my sister Carol Koltz, my sister-in-law Toni Burbank, and all the Maxwells, Grinnens, and Michaleks.

Finally, let me give a special note of thanks to my wife, Martha Michalek, who has supported me in so many ways, both small and large, that it's impossible to express their cumulative power. Quite simply, this book wouldn't have happened without her.

Preface

The Sugarman Prophecy

Nothing in my life ever prepared me to have diabetes.

I knew this by the time I reported to the health center at the University of Massachusetts-Amherst on a dreary day in March of 1996 to find out how to prick my fingertips and take the blood-sugar tests that would become my whole point of reference.

I had been diagnosed with adult-onset, non-insulin-dependent, type 2 diabetes about ten days before, and I was just beginning to accept the reality of this sweet kiss of death.

Leaning against the check-in desk was an older African-American man wearing faded overalls and a whimsical expression, someone who was obviously here for the same reason I was. Our group orientation session with a nurse was part of the treatment process for all recently diagnosed people with diabetes.

The man's appearance struck me instantly, as if some old-time Southern blues singer, some Muddy Waters or Leadbelly or Blind Lemon, had jetted through a time warp into our lily-white New England college town.

While I identified myself to the nurse, the man continued to eye me with a look of kindly good humor. Then I realized he was about to strike up a conversation. There was a moment of pregnant silence as I asked myself the first question I always pose about all chance encounters with strangers. Is this going to be embarrassing?

"So," he finally said. "You're a sugarman just like me."

It took me several moments to take in the significance of this droll remark: that I was entering a new community made up of people with diabetes, that we were all in this together, and that there was even a clever nickname attached to the membership. The very sound tasted like honey on my tongue. Sugarman. Sugarwoman. Sugarpeople.

"Yipes," I remember thinking, as if I were some comic-book character with emotions expressed in dialog balloons. Then I began to laugh, for the first time since diabetes had changed my life. It was a deep laugh that felt like whitewater rushing over a dam and aerating in bright, clean air.

The Ability to Whine
Intellectually

Since being diagnosed with diabetes, I had been feeling sorry for myself in an elaborate way. One of the wonders of higher education is that it confers the ability to whine intellectually. All my time as a student and employee on college campuses, some 20 years, had taught me to camouflage sniveling with the high-tone language of angst. Now, with one witty observation, a sugarman from out of nowhere made me understand what a jerk I'd been with my self-pity. He gave me the sudden distance that only humor can bring to any serious business.

In many ways, this chance encounter with the sugarman was the defining moment of my life. Eventually, diabetes would completely transform me from what poet T.S. Eliot called a hollow man, suffering all the bouts of meaninglessness and dissatisfaction native to modern society, into a sugarman, infused with a new kind of sweetness that would fill my soul.

It was as if that fanciful man at the health center were some kind of messenger, some kind of apparition, sent to give me a wake-up call. In many ways, I suppose, such messages are the purpose of every encounter every day, if only we had the presence of mind to stop, look, and listen. Perhaps I'd been waiting all my life for this kind of vision to shake me up.

"To know the sweetness of the Infinite within us," said 15th-century mystic Nicholas of Cusa, "that is the cause, the reason, the purpose, the only purpose of our being."

The infinite effect of my diabetes would be what mystics sometimes call a "locution," a disembodied voice delivering an occult message in the manner of some heavenly figure from a beatific experience, some spirit from a Shakespearean tragedy, or some hallucination in a schizophrenic episode. By their very nature, all locutions work through shock value, scaring the hell out of us and sending us scurrying along the path of righteousness.

In the case of my own locution, the shock being delivered would prove to be a kind of diabetic shock.

I couldn't have known it at the moment, but my own locution set off a coming revolution deep within my psyche. It would not only overturn the physical makeup of my body, but the psychological regime of my mind.

God Has No Religion

The story I am about to tell is a very personal account of how I am trying to face the most serious crisis of my life. It is the story of my resurrection from a life without any particular meaning and my rebirth into a new "state of grace," as religious doctrine would phrase my fresh outlook on existence.

Not being a religious person myself, I feel quite uncomfortable with the dogma created by most religions. As Mahatma Gandhi said, "God has no religion."

My journey toward understanding would
become more of a diabetic than a religious pilgrimage.
Still, in my own agnostic and blundering way, I would
soon begin shambling toward Canaan. Diabetes would
inspire me to find the deeper currents of spirituality
that were coursing through my arteries, along with the
sickly-sweet baptism of my new disease. It would be no
great exaggeration to call diabetes a spiritual experience, in much the same vein as a bar mitzvah, a sacrament, or the moment of enlightenment.

The challenge of diabetes, as I am discovering, is
not so much physical as metaphysical. Dealing with
diabetes in the physical sense is rather routine: taking
care of diet, exercising regularly, paying attention to
the warning signs given by my body, and living the
kind of healthy lifestyle that everyone ought to practice
anyway. But dealing with diabetes in the emotional and
spiritual sense is the most challenging and transforming experience of my days on earth.

My fateful meeting with diabetes often reminds
me of the ancient Chinese character for crisis, a graceful
nest of brush strokes, space, and symbolism that combines the elements of both challenge and opportunity.
Certainly all that symbolism, fraught with both its per-
ils and its potential, was present in the way I was forced
to deal with the sugar running amuck in my circulatory
system.

The dual nature of my own crisis eventually
turned me from a rudderless soul into a person with a
strict sense of mission. Turned me from a materialist
into a contemplative. From a shallow fellow into some-

one aware of life's deeper wellsprings. From an escapist into a realist. From an atheist into a believer in the dizzying intelligence of nature. From a hollow man into a sugarman.

Managing my blood sugar has really become a symbol for managing my emotions, managing my spirituality, managing my meaningfulness, managing my philosophy, managing my creativity. These are the elements of diabetes I want to convey to you.

This book is essentially about spiritual transformation. But in the sense that I am neither religious in any way, nor a theist in the traditional way, I need to define for you the kind of spirituality I practice in my own life.

I fully recognize that faith is a very personal form of hope that means something different to each human being. Though I respect and admire many kinds of spiritual and religious belief, I have never felt at home in any organized religion. In my case, spirituality is basically a communion with the intelligence of nature. It is a way to appreciate the unearthly beauty of the universe, the supernatural order of creation, and the meaningfulness of my own life, which, in retrospect, seems to have taken a course dictated by intellect far beyond my comprehension.

To me, spirituality is a state of optimism, purpose, tolerance, compassion, acceptance, and truthfulness that gives direction to my life and shapes my future. To my mind, the power and genius of the cosmos itself is the deity I recognize as my own, and the search for my true inner self (my immortal soul, if you will) is the form my worship takes.

One's Life, One's Soul, One's Health, One's Future

As you read the following pages, I want you to see through my own eyes the transforming quality diabetes can have on one's life, one's soul, one's health, one's future. I want you to live my own story and other diabetic stories to see how this transformation can take place. I want you to read the comments of medical professionals about the power of metaphysics and soul-searching as they influence blood-sugar maintenance and health in general. And, finally, I want you to consider my own modest example of spiritual practice as a touchstone in your own soul-search for meaning, peace of mind, and a healthier tomorrow.

I have organized *Zen and the Art of Diabetes Maintenance* into three parts that I hope will take you logically and, more or less, painlessly through the above process:

- Part 1, Shambling Toward Canaan, which will tell the personal story of how diabetes transformed my life and supercharged my spirituality
- Part 2, Insulin for the Soul, which will explore the medical benefits of spirituality as it influences health, and will tell the true stories of people with diabetes who were transformed spiritually and physically by diabetes
- Part 3, Zen and the Art of Diabetes Maintenance, which will suggest seven simple

practices that can serve as a spiritual guide for people with diabetes while striving for total health of mind and body

The Secret God Behind the Gods

One word of qualification about this book: *Zen and the Art of Diabetes Maintenance* is meant as a whimsical, tongue-in-cheek title. In no way am I trying to pass myself off as an expert on Zen, on Buddhism, or on any other philosophy. To paraphrase the wonderful lyric of singer-composer Joan Osborne, I'm just a slob like all of us; a slob who's learned a thing or two about the spiritual side of managing diabetes. I'd like to pass it along to you.

My book carries a universal message to people with diabetes everywhere. Listen to the life force of your innermost self, for in your soul lies the answer to every trial and tribulation. In the process, you might even find the answers to a lot of mysteries you didn't even know you were aching to solve.

Each in his or her own way, we are all searching for the "secret god behind the gods," as Ralph Waldo Emerson once described his transcendental philosophy. We are all looking for that "poem in the heart of things," which poet Wallace Stevens was searching for in each of his verses. In my case, diabetes was the oracle that alerted me to these mystic possibilities.

In its most basic sense, this book is the story of a "conversion," that dry-sounding term religion often uses to express the fury, pandemonium, and disaster needed to overcome any loss of faith. My own conversion through an angel of death called diabetes took a lifetime of mistakes, a mortal threat to my health and well-being, a confrontation with the most dangerous foe I've ever faced, and a fateful meeting with an unlikely prophet who would baptize me as a sugarman, just like him.

All these factors conspired to teach me one key lesson about the person I used to be. To quote the insightful language of Pogo, that philosophical swamp creature who regularly appeared in comic strips of yesteryear:

"I have met the enemy, and he was me."

PART one

Shambling Toward Canaan

*How Diabetes
Transformed
My Life*

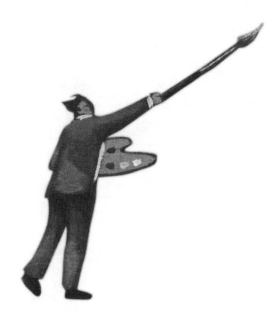

Property of the
Mir Space Station
The Day I Learned I Had Diabetes

The telephone has become so ordinary an instrument of communication, so humdrum a miracle of electronics, that nobody expects it to deliver heavenly messages that really ought to be carved on stone tablets. If Moses had heard a disembodied voice speaking to him through such a peculiar object as a telephone, he might have fallen to his knees and prayed. But brought up in an age of mass-produced miracles, I was barely aware of the cosmic messenger speaking from the other end of the line.

"Can I talk to Charles Creekmore please?"

"Speaking."

"Mr. Creekmore," the crisp young female voice said, "I'm calling from Dr. Morgan's office."

"Yes?"

"The doctor was wondering if you could come to the health center at two o'clock this afternoon."

"I guess so. But what about?"

"Well, some abnormalities have shown up in your blood tests from last week."

"Abnormalities?"

"Yes, in your glucose readings."

"My what?"

"Your fasting blood-sugar levels."

"I don't under. . ."

"I think it would be better if Dr. Morgan described the problem himself."

Understanding Life Backwards

And so it began. Or maybe I should say, and so it ended. "Life can only be understood backwards," Danish philosopher and theologian Søren Kierkegaard once observed, "but it must be lived forwards."

With the benefit of backwards thinking, I now understand the exact beginning of this story, which not by coincidence marked the exact ending of my previous life. With hindsight, I now see that the heavens cracked open like the jaws of a whale and spit me out through the jack of a Bell telephone wire. The herald bringing my fate came to me as a disembodied female voice reluctant to break the bad news all in one bolt of lightning.

I suppose it's a fitting comment on the nature of contemporary life that harbingers come wrapped, not in bright auras and feathery pinions, but in electronic circuits and plastic receivers.

By chance, a few minutes after the disturbing call from Dr. Morgan's office, I found myself staring at a note printed by some wag in my office building at the University of Massachusetts in Amherst. The mock notice was taped to our temperamental copy machine, which regularly flashed the "paper jam" sign on its little digital face.

"Property of the Mir Space Station," the note read.

That message might have described my whole life, as if some high school prankster had slapped this note on my back 40 years before and I had been walking around like that ever since. As I would soon come to understand, the curse of the Mir Space Station, that heavenly accident in search of an orbit in happenstance, is what my own diabetes was all about. It was a secret malfunction in either my pancreas or the very chemistry of my cells waiting all my life for a chance to go wrong.

The Hack Writer in Residence

Unaware of the epiphany represented by that first telephone conversation with Dr. Morgan's receptionist, I remember feeling little more anxiety than if I'd just been informed of an ulcer. I gave almost no thought to the source of this communication, my own bloodstream, whose veins and arteries were carrying a deadly sweetness to every tissue, organ, and nerve inside my anatomy. Likewise, I carefully ignored the possible death sentence I'd just been handed by a judge as enigmatic as death itself.

I passed the time before my appointment with Dr. Morgan by carrying out the pedestrian duties of my job at UMass, where I was gainfully underemployed in a position I often referred to as the Hack Writer in Residence. My real title was Senior Writer, but I had gradually come to the conclusion that the "senior" in that name pertained more to my age than my status. In that capacity, I wrote speeches for our highly articulate chancellor, Dr. David Scott, who used my scribbles as what he called "inspiration" for his own spontaneous remarks. My own carefully crafted doggerel rarely saw the light of day. He liked my jokes, though, and often employed my one-liners to punctuate his own oratory. Seen in that light, I was basically the chancellor's gag writer.

It was also my job to cobble together the rhetoric needed for academic ceremonies taking place each year at the university, a task that included writing the speeches, scripts, award certificates, and honorary-degree citations given at convocations, galas, and commencements.

In other words, my employment consisted mainly of creating the white noise for all the main events on campus.

On this prophetic day I busied myself working on a chancellor's speech for the upcoming dedication of our new polymer science building, confident as usual that I could say whatever I damn well pleased on paper, for my actual words would never be spoken into any microphone at any real event. My mission, in this case, was simply to jostle the chancellor's sensibilities into saying what he would say anyway.

My Pancreas Cannibalizing Itself

It was a typical March day in New England, full of the bluster and brightness of weathery change. As I made my way cross-campus to the health center, my mind was more on the thermodynamics of the wind bustling up my coat than the medical dynamics of sugar rushing through my internal rivers.

Then I felt something shiver through me as I trudged through the windy canyon created by our Fine Arts Center, a great slab of artificial cliffs shaped, as some say, to resemble a concrete piano. A troubling thought quivered down my spine like a bad key vibrating. I remembered the one medical emergency I'd ever suffered, some 18 years before, when a sado-masochistic love affair, a urinary-tract infection, a prescription of tetracycline, and my own escapist attitude had all somehow conspired to bring on an acute case of pancreatitis that almost killed me.

It had been a life-threatening condition created by the digestive enzymes secreted from my pancreas surrounding the organ itself and cannibalizing its own flesh. My former doctor had warned me that one long-term consequence of pancreatitis might be diabetes.

But in my typical fashion, I had ignored his prediction in the hopes that simple forgetfulness could serve as my elixir.

As I sat in the waiting room of the health center—full of the usual posters about lower-back pain, weight control, and genital herpes—I noticed my hands and arm pits growing clammy, as if my body were listening to some voice that my mind could not yet sense. Why does perception so often work this way, with the extra-sensory outracing the sensory to the brain?

Dr. Warren Morgan, my primary physician, was a tall, slightly shy, youthful-looking man with a kindly face and the sincere eyes of someone who believes devoutly in what he does. He might have been a Liberation Theologist, a Greenpeace demonstrator, or a Red Cross relief worker. In addition to the usual medical paraphernalia decorating his office, there were pictures of his loved ones framed and positioned with the care of a dedicated family man.

Though I knew him only slightly, I knew him well enough to grasp the gravity of my situation by the way he began our conversation.

"I'm not going to lie to you," he said.

"Okay."

"It seems your lab report has come back with a fasting blood-glucose level of 375 mg/dl."

"I'm sorry, doctor. That figure means nothing to me."

"Your blood sugar is nearly four times higher than normal. If this is an accurate lab report, the chances are pretty fair you've developed a diabetic condition."

I watched him with the part of my consciousness that protects against swift jolts of bad news with doubt and befuddlement.

"But labs sometimes get it wrong," he said. "And so do all the rest of us in the medical community. We're going to do some additional blood tests to make sure."

Even as he said this, however, I knew it wasn't so. The lab didn't get it wrong, and Dr. Morgan was simply acting like a careful and thorough professional. It was beginning to sink in that something terrible was happening to my body; something that, unlike most realities in my life, I couldn't run away from. Something that I couldn't ignore.

Where Everyone's Fear of Death Resides

"I'm going to level with you," Dr. Morgan continued. "Diabetes is a very serious condition. One of the more serious problems that anyone can develop. But it's also a condition that you can control. Every person with diabetes has the ability to manage the future. It doesn't have to end in the complications you've heard about."

"I have to confess," I said, "I don't have any idea what complications you mean."

"Let me sum it up this way. If left unchecked, excess blood sugar can eventually impair almost every system in the body. But if you manage it properly, you can be as long-lived and healthy as anyone else. Maybe even more so. We're going to teach you how to do that. To manage your blood sugar."

"How?"

"First, we're going to do some more tests to confirm if the initial ones were accurate. If they were, we'll want to determine whether you can manage your blood sugar with diet and exercise. Or, if that doesn't work out, you might need insulin injections or oral medication to help control your glucose levels. Meanwhile, my nurse will make an appointment for you with our nutritionist. We'll also send you to someone who'll teach you how to take your own blood-sugar readings. The best tactic for dealing with diabetes is education, monitoring, and proper management."

"And if I don't do any of that?"

His gaze, staring into the far blacks of my pupils, where everyone's fear of death resides, revealed more than the hard facts he didn't want to spell out this early in the treatment.

"I'll give you some material to read," he said.

The pamphlets he handed me were composed in that bland style used by medical bulletins to teach people about their worst fears. I suspect these publications are always written in such a detached way because, by dehumanizing the fearful message they bring, their language can demystify the horror they describe.

A quick glance at the literature gave me a laundry list of reasons why I might not reach a ripe old age. Or if I did, I wouldn't like it. Diabetic shock, seizures, coma, nerve damage, infection, kidney failure, blindness, heart attack, stroke, coronary disease, gangrene, amputation: It was a litany of pain, distress, and deadliness that turned aging into a mine field of hidden terrors.

The Importance of What Doesn't Happen

Dr. Morgan's approach was obvious. He was upbeat and frank, encouraging me to manage my blood sugar competently and informing me why this process was necessary. But he didn't barrage me with so many horror stories that I became too discouraged to face my situation. His was the appropriate professional response to my condition.

But as a journalist, I have long since learned the importance of what doesn't happen or isn't said in any story; for that which doesn't occur surrounds that which does and forms its boundaries. I sensed what Dr. Morgan wasn't saying. Now the truth in absentia scared the hell out of me.

It was at this moment, sitting in Dr. Morgan's office as he scribbled information in my medical record, that I recalled where I'd seen his penetrating gaze before. It was during the spring of 1979, as I hovered near death in the intensive care unit with my case of pancreatitis. All the friends and loved ones stopping by my bedside projected that same dark cast from the eyes, the knowing and sympathetic gaze of J. Alfred Prufrock's eternal footman.

"You can tell a lot about a person by the enemies he keeps," Sherlock Holmes had once said to Dr. Watson about the elusive villain, Professor Moriarity. By that same token, you can tell a lot about people by the diseases they keep.

I was about to meet my own Professor Moriarity in the brilliant disguise of diabetes, and whatever future I possessed would be decided by whether I could outwit him or not.

Or more importantly, whether I could understand him or not.

The Accidental Monk

My Reckless History

At the age of 50, I was little more prepared for diabetes than for a locution from the heavens. I had led an interesting, if ill-advised, life as a writer and "long-distance runner" in its every connotation. Almost 30 years before diabetes, my then father-in-law had astutely summed up my personality by nicknaming me "The Freelancer."

In his zeal to express how unworthy I was to marry his daughter, he had correctly figured out that I was not the sort to be connected to anyone, anything, or anywhere for very long. I was a freelancer in every way, as I eventually proved by leaving his daughter after a stormy marriage.

Pointedly enough, my confrontation with diabetes occurred almost 20 years to the day after I divorced my first wife and within weeks after I became engaged to my second. Martha, my fiancée, was the "good woman"—the decent, smart, and true-hearted woman—all my close friends had always said I needed. With her quiet, strong, and kindly influence came the stability that I had not only lacked for my entire life, but had actively avoided.

Now I was surprised to learn that part of my evolving stability was about to be administered by something even more elusive than love. Just to make certain my staying power took hold, the universal forces that control existence were joining me in a new kind of wedlock, in sickness and in health, to love and to cherish, till death do us part.

This other lover's knot was called diabetes.

My Vagabond Nature

There was good enough reason for my vagabond nature. I grew up in east Texas with a gift for running that would spread to many facets of my life.

My father was a pilot who died in an airliner disaster in 1947, when I was two. After my mother remarried in 1952, my step-father, an ex-Marine, proved to be a charming but troubled man whose idea of family life was boot camp at Paris Island. He was "The Great Santini" in the flesh. I spent much of my childhood standing at attention, doing chores with minute precision, learning the hard knocks of Marine Corps discipline, and enduring the humiliation that is any draftee's lot.

I also found out the hard way what every military brat knows about the Corps: Once a Marine, always a Marine. *Semper fidelis.* Ten years of tough love imbued me with a fierce hatred of authority, an aching inferiority complex, an addiction to adventure, and an obsession with running from reality.

By the time my family moved to northern New Jersey in the late 1950s, I was fast enough to excel as a track and field athlete at my local high school, Bergen Catholic, where I won numerous county, state, and regional medals as a quarter-miler and relay anchorman. Then a pulled hamstring muscle at the Bergen County Championships in 1963 changed my life in many unpredictable ways.

The force of that beefy muscle complex snapping shot me straight up in the air, as if my body were propelled by a huge, broken rubberband. By the time I landed a split-second later, this acute muscle tear had changed me from an athlete into a writer. No longer able to obsess about my track career, which came to an end as I lay writhing on the cinders of the Northern Valley Regional High School track, I soon turned to another talent, as yet undiscovered, that would drive my entire future—the ability to turn a phrase.

Great Moments of Truth

That muscle pull would become one of several great moments of truth, which seemed to happen to me once every decade. The first was my father's airliner death in 1947, the second my mother's re-marriage in the 1950s. Another was this track injury in the 1960s. Next came my bout with pancreatitis at the close of the 1970s. My wake-up call for the 1980s was a mystical occurrence at a Trappist monastery, as you will soon read. And the defining event of the 1990s, and perhaps my whole life, was the onset of diabetes.

Each of these momentous events altered me quite completely, and quite against my will, in much the same way that matter is turned into energy by brute physical force. This is the kind of pandemonium and blood-letting it takes to turn faithless people such as myself into what the Sufis call "The Changed Ones."

After that muscle tear ended all my athletic dreams, I spent the next 30 years parlaying my matching gifts for speed and wit into a writing career and lifestyle; except now I was no longer running from lean sprinters as before, but from a reality I couldn't face.

I became a widely published poet, fiction writer, and journalist whose freelance assignments and jobs took me all over the world. I also served as a volunteer for VISTA, the Peace Corps, and the United Nations, and signed on as a member of a biological expedition tracking monarch butterflies to their wintering sites in central Mexico. In the down time between such adventures, I worked as a reporter on three newspapers, a wordsmith at UMass, Amherst College, and Washington University, and a science writer for the United Nations Environment Programme in Nairobi, Kenya.

Meanwhile, having permanently scarred the power muscles needed for sprinting, I turned into an avid long-distance runner, a dirty little habit I've now practiced religiously for 40 years.

In a way, running kept me sane; but by serving as my escape valve, it also kept me from concentrating on the deeper questions that every life well-lived must produce. What is the meaning of existence? Why are we here? What is the real nature, the deeper reality, of that cliché we have made of God? What is my ultimate purpose in the scheme of things? What must I do to give myself meaning, satisfaction, and peace of mind?

Ignoring these questions for so long was no easy task. I lived by a creed that for many years I kept taped over the keyboard of my manual typewriter. It read: "Think Shallow."

You're a Puer Aeternus, Aren't You?

I began to sense the significance of all life's unanswered questions during one of my aforementioned moments of truth; this one in 1989, while I was making an eight-month-long retreat to a place where staying power, devotion, and the contemplation of existential mysteries was a way of life. I'd arranged to live as a long-term visitor at a Trappist monastery in northern California during the throes of a nervous breakdown, caused, in effect, by three decades of nonstop running, as I wandered willy-nilly from one journalistic gig to the next.

Even though at the time I practiced a faithless form of agnosticism with absolutely no purpose, my choice to stay in a monastery was no act of serendipity. I had recently returned from Nairobi, working for the

UN. At the age of 44, I found myself with no real goals, no definable philosophy, no hope for the future, and no clue about what to do now. My only *raison d'être* was looking for the next adventure, which I'd currently found in an impossible love affair. The whole situation brought my life to a boil with a sense of alienation and meaninglessness that had been simmering for decades. It also turned me into a mental wreck.

That emotional breakdown, I now understand, was a gift, given by an intellect beyond the pale of my knowledge as a way to slow down my runaway life and piece it back together. Somehow, even in my harried state, I intuited that mine was not a crisis of the mind, but of the spirit.

As a last resort, I arranged with the abbot to stay at his monastery in exchange for working around the grounds. He was a good man, who must have seen the desperation in my eyes, and must have sensed why I'd really come to his cloister. I was here on some spiritual quest beyond my ability to explain. I spent my time at the abbey in work and meditation and contemplation, as I tried to figure out where my existence had all gone wrong.

The unexamined part of my life may have started shining through on a warm autumn evening while I was living the life of an accidental monk. On this particular night, I was eating dinner in the guest dining room when a kindred stranger peered across the table at me with some amount of curiosity. He watched me in much the same way, I now see in retrospect, as that sugarman would regard me years later at the UMass Health Center—with the kindly eyes of a prophet.

"You're a *puer aeternus*, aren't you?" the stranger opened our conversation.

"A what?" I said.

"That's Latin for eternal boy. It's one of Jung's concepts, and I can see it in your eyes. I'm a *puer* myself."

Sure enough, as I gazed into the man's eyes, they reflected my own, looking like he had just stolen fire from the gods and was searching for someone to hand it to.

During the next two hours, which we spent strolling through the eventide and cricket throb of the monastery grounds, my new friend described my life in accurate detail, simply by recounting his own: the adventure; the risk-taking; the regular movements from job to job and place to place; the passionate, short-lived romances that burned themselves out almost as quickly as they began.

"You see," he said, "I've spent my whole life questing after the perfect woman. I was looking for the Blessed Virgin Mary in every woman I loved. And as soon as I found she wasn't the saint I envisioned, then I had to leave and go somewhere else. I guess my search is what brings me here. What better place to find the mother of God than a monastery?"

Time Wounds All Heels

Through this meeting and many other small epiphanies at the monastery, I arrived at a troubling revelation about myself. I was addicted to moving from

place to place and woman to woman. I was both a
geographic and a romantic junky.

If ever I would succeed in coming to grips with
the essence of my life, the purpose of my being, I would
have to come home to myself. I would have to come
home to the person inside and stay there. All my
movement, all my adventure, had all gone for naught.
With all my feverish changes, all my time on the road,
I had accomplished nothing of lasting importance,
written nothing of permanent value, left nothing of
eternal worth, touched no one in an undying way.

In many ways, I was the personification of the
word "quixotic." Like Don Quixote, I was a knight
errant, with the emphasis on *errant*. During the
previous 25 years, I had wandered the world searching
for illusions such as fame, excitement, adventure, and
the perfect love. I had been dreaming the impossible
dream. I was Quixote chasing after a Dulcinea who
didn't even exist. Worst of all, I viewed this romantic
adventure as something holy, when in reality I was
questing in a fool's paradise.

As the master of my illusions, I had yet to
acknowledge that I was solely responsible for my own
deluded actions. Such personal responsibility is one
idea found in karma, that complex Eastern concept
of universal comeuppance that, in typical Western
fashion, I had once seen condensed into the flippant
language of a bumper sticker:

"Time Wounds All Heels."

With my live-for-today philosophy, I continued
to be wounded time and time again by the bad karma
of my past. In the process, I had never stopped to face

the reality of my own immaturity, embodied in my *puer aeternus* complex.

Psychologist Carl Jung once defined the key dilemma of any *puer aeternus*: either a person must begin the difficult quest for meaning and understanding during the process of maturation, or else that person will become nothing more than "an applauder of the past, an eternal adolescent—lamentable substitutes for the illumination of the self."

It was shortly after leaving the monastery that I moved back to western Massachusetts, met Martha, and began to find myself.

Rabbi Seymour Siegel once expressed the longing that ailed me better than I ever could: "In everyone's heart stirs a great homesickness."

At the monastery, I began to dissolve my quixotic illusions, and now I was ready for the next step in my evolution: creating the spiritual life that would become my psychic home. The rest of this book is the story of how a spiritual guru called diabetes helped me cure the great homesickness in my own heart, and how, by extension, it can help you cure the great homesickness in yours.

If my whole book could be distilled into one all-encompassing word, I would hope it might be the ever-hopeful, always joyful idea of "homecoming." The home, in this case, is that feathery, wise, and luminous tongue of fire called the self, which each of us carries inside wherever we go.

That's what diabetes was about to help me find.

Down and Out in Provincetown

A Period of Adjustment to
My New Condition

Whenever I look back on my first week as a guy newly diagnosed with diabetes, after Dr. Morgan gave me the bad news at the UMass health center, I always think of actress Isabella Rossellini. She was the Muse, made from oil paint and canvas, who presided over my initial, bumbling efforts as a person coping with diabetes.

At the time of my diagnosis, my newly betrothed Martha and I had already scheduled our yearly vacation on Cape Cod for the upcoming week. We decided to forge ahead with our plans in the hope that Cape Cod would prove a good place to take stock of diabetes and consider how it would affect our lives together.

Under normal circumstances, we would have stayed at one of the less expensive guest houses on the

Cape, considering that Hack Writers in Residence have never rated among the most well-paid employees of the state university system.

Instead, we decided to splurge, mainly because I felt as though a black hole had settled in my endocrine system. I suppose we were falling back on the traditional solution of Americans for any depression, whether it be personal or national in nature—gross overspending.

We checked into an atmospheric waterfront cottage colony in the quiet West End of Provincetown, a place that was way above our means and way over our budget. While the manager was showing us around our charming two-story cottage, Martha and I both froze in our tracks at the foot of the stairs. Peering up the steps, we were mesmerized by a large, brutally rendered portrait hung above the stairwell. The oil painting in question undoubtedly pictured Isabella Rossellini, but in some kind of altered state. The portrait seemed to be done, whether intentionally or not, in a kind of expressionist style that gave symbolic substance to the inner disturbances of the subject. It was as if the elegant star were possessed by something unmentionable.

Whatever vision had been conjured in the mind of the deeply disturbed artist, the icon on this canvas was in dire need of either an antacid or an exorcist.

Martha and I stared for several seconds at the portrait's brooding colors and the distracted expression on the celebrity's face, as though she had been conjured up as a 17th-century resident of Salem on trial for witchery.

"Isn't she lovely?" said the manager.

"Words can't express it," I said.

"She was done by a local artist, you know, when she was on location for *Tough Guys Don't Dance.*"

"It's uncanny," said Martha.

"Isabella gave it to us right before she left," the manager bragged.

"How generous," I observed, trying to avoid the portrait's ravaged eyes.

"So we hung it here," said the manager, "because this was the cottage where she stayed."

"Lucky us," I said.

Gazing into the Gaping Maw of Indigestion

If it is true, as Oscar Wilde's saying goes, that God punishes sinners by giving them what they pray for, then the converse must also be true. What God curses us with often turns out to be a blessing in disguise.

This paradox would soon be verified by both my diabetes and my brush with Isabella Rossellini's woebegone portrait. In both cases, God's blessings were very well disguised.

That week in the Rossellini cottage must certainly have been the darkest vacation I would ever spend, as I was reminded each time I trudged up those steps and found myself gazing into the gaping maw of Isabella's indigestion.

The first problem I needed to face in Provincetown was my limited education about diabetic nutrition, a little knowledge that was about to become a dangerous thing, at least to my sense of taste.

The nutritionist at UMass had sent me on what would prove to be a fool's errand. She had wanted me to spend the week of my vacation experimenting with a diet that was basically fit for termites. The purpose, of course, was to find out how much effect a Spartan diet would exert on my blood sugar. It would be the key factor for determining whether or not Dr. Morgan would need to prescribe a diabetes medication.

Thus, we stocked our little overpriced kitchen with a motley assortment of foodstuff based on my half-hour crash course in diabetic nutrition and my half-baked notion of what the nutritionist had told me. As I understood my mission, I was to lay off carbohydrates entirely. Sugar, needless to say, was out. Lean meat, in small portions, was acceptable, though frowned upon. Fish, which I'd always detested because of the tiny bones, was suggested as my main source of protein. I was also allowed ample amounts of dietetic sweets, which I soon found was like quenching a roaring thirst with salt water.

What was left to form the bulk of my diet were various vegetables, which I had always regarded in much the same way college freshmen regard their required courses.

After returning from the supermarket and surveying the meager pickings available to me, I recalled the griping of a diabetic friend of mine about the diet he was forced to adopt.

"Rabbit food," he called it.

Drowning in My
Own Bloodstream

March on the Cape is always a mixed bag.
The weather alternates between drizzly dreariness,
mindful of those places on earth with the highest
suicide rates, and luke-warm sunniness, which teases
those of us who long for something a little more
Mediterranean. Not unlike the portrait hanging at
the top of the staircase, the weather during this
particular week seemed to reflect the desolation of
my own soul.

I remember sitting alone in the upstairs
bedroom, after having run the rapids of Isabella's
turbulent gaze on the stairs, and feeling the whole river
of my diabetes washing over me. Through my window,
Provincetown harbor appeared stark and colorless. So
did my future.

I felt like a man drowning in his own bloodstream.

I was buffeted by waves of emotion. I ran the
whole gauntlet of emotions that most people with
diabetes suffer soon after their initial diagnosis: anger,
horror, denial, despair, and that old standby, self-pity.
There was also rage, naturally. Every person with
diabetes feels rage at the universe for the bad hand
being dealt. Then there was a vague feeling of guilt,
spawned no doubt by my Catholic upbringing. What
had I done to deserve all this? I must have committed
unspeakable acts of impurity to be sentenced to such a
punishment.

After I had finished scourging myself for every
moment of intemperance or misdemeanor in my past,

that's when I took a cruise in my own mental lifeboat, which I had long ago christened the "Hari-kari."

For my whole adulthood, I'd played a little mind game with myself as a way of fending off my worst fears. If things got too bad, or so I would tell myself, I'd simply do myself in. I suspect this suicidal mindset was really my substitute for belief in a supreme deity, an afterlife, or any kind of spiritual salvation. Having little in the way of a spiritual life, I had adopted suicide as my religion. With nothing to elevate myself above the frightening appearances of hard reality, I reasoned that a merciful death might be the only *deus ex machina* available to save face in the final act of my life. It was my only means, as I viewed it, of gaining any control over the slings and arrows of outrageous fortune.

Though I had never actually tried to commit suicide, I had always found that wallowing in the possibilities acted as a kind of sacrament to bless my state of depression. Though this exercise in self-pity seems almost comical as I look back on it now, a very real life-and-death struggle was taking place. I was asking myself the ultimate existential question about diabetes. How much can I take, and how much not?

Thus, brooding by myself as I watched the gray clouds moping outside my widow, I worked like an accountant over his ledger. In this instance, I was calculating a list of diabetic complications I couldn't handle, now or ever. The inventory included stroke, paralysis, amputation, blindness, any terminal disease, excessive pain, and simple hopelessness.

Engaged in this unhealthy activity, I sat in that upstairs bedroom for what seemed like hours, feeling as Isabella must have felt while sitting for her expressionist painting—like a subject waiting to be executed.

The Tyranny of Carrot Juice, Celery, and Dietary Eskimo Pies

If there was madness to my method, I gradually realized there was also method to my madness.

Each new experience tainted with diabetes, as I would find out, was part of a learning curve whose trajectory would sail me past all my anger and hurt into a quiet place where I could absorb the lessons this experience had to teach.

For example, there was my first night dining out as a person with diabetes. Martha and I ate at an atmospheric Provincetown bistro named Nappi's, which had always been our favorite haunt on the Cape. A quick glance at the menu convinced me I couldn't order any of my usual high-carbo, high-calorie favorites because they would bust my diet. So, instead, I went where no Creekmore had ever gone before. I ordered a Brazilian seafood dish, substituting spicy condiments and vegetables for the banana fritters, hot rolls, and rice I really craved.

What I discovered, to my astonishment, was how the exotic tastes and wholesome ingredients delighted my palate. After that night, I began to take great pleasure in cuisines and food groups I would never have entertained, much less savored, in the past.

This newfound enjoyment of unlikely foods proved a revelation to me, even though I *did* spend much of that vacation back at the Rossellini cottage, standing and staring forlornly into the fridge and suffering the tyranny of carrot juice, celery, and dietary Eskimo Pies.

Drafted into Spiritual Boot Camp

One drizzly afternoon in Provincetown, Martha and I passed a few hours filling out the invitations to our wedding, which was then about three months away. Somehow, this boring exercise in propriety taught me a lasting lesson about staying power and commitment.

During the course of that afternoon, scribbling out salutations and addresses, the idea first occurred to me, as I wrote earlier in the book, that I was now betrothed in more ways than one. The good news was my upcoming marriage to Martha, the kind of relationship I had needed for a very long time. The bad news was my engagement to a permanent medical condition, which, strange as it sounds, I also needed in some way.

How is it possible that anyone could need anything as potentially destructive as diabetes?

While I spent that afternoon at the chore of writing wedding invitations, I began to understand how diabetes was beginning to train me in a new set of abilities I had never possessed:

- responsibility to oneself, one's body, and one's spirit

- enough self-discipline to perform the everyday tasks, the daily grind, that nobody likes doing
- the skills necessary for self-examination, in both the physical and emotional senses
- the perseverance needed for carrying on a healthy long-term regimen
- attention to the small details that make such a vital difference to one's health over the course of a lifetime
- the compassionate traits of tolerance, good will, and patience, which are the bellwether attitudes needed for dealing with any chronic illness

It was as though I were sitting for a portrait, and the painter was amplifying my likeness with a set of new virtues. The painter, in this case, was diabetes.

But, with the value added by diabetes came the responsibility of putting my new virtues into action. What I was discovering about diabetes was the same thing I had discovered about the art of writing, nearly a quarter-century before: It takes a hell of a lot of organization and hard work.

None of my friends, family, and loved ones, when they received those wedding invitations scrawled in my own unsteady hand, could have realized that each note was really a brush stroke in the whole new design for my life, one based on spiritual structure and discipline. None of them could have known I was being re-painted, moment by moment, and daub by daub.

March Madness

I made another discovery during that stay in the Rossellini cottage. It amounted to my own brand of "March Madness," that TV moniker for the NCAA Basketball Tournament.

Nineteen-Ninety-Six happened to be the year when the UMass basketball squad had its best season ever. A young firebrand named John Calipari, in his very first head-coaching assignment, had transformed the UMass basketball program from one of the worst in all Division I, to one of the best. And, that week in Provincetown, Martha and I saw Calipari's team enjoy its finest hour on national TV during the NCAA Tournament.

Perhaps, by this point in my emotional week, every event was taking on symbolic meaning, and every moment was waxing monumental. I don't know. But, as we sat in our exorbitant little rented living room, scrutinized by the mournful gaze of Isabella Rossellini at the top of the stairs, and watched the scrappy UMass team win a hard-fought game against Georgetown to qualify for the Final Four, I was inspired in my own rite.

Seemingly, Coach Cal had sculpted this team from his own willpower. He had infused these young players with the spirit of his own slogan: "Refuse to Lose." As hokey as this saying had seemed to me over the past few years, now that spirit was being absorbed into my very cells as I watched UMass players fighting ruthlessly over every free ball and defending feistily against every Georgetown shot.

I am reminded of a landfill company that had recycled Coach Cal's slogan on all its garbage trucks. "Refuse to Lose," said the trucks, altering the whole meaning of the slogan by simply changing the first word from a verb to a noun.

In a like manner, I had been recycled by diabetes. It had changed my syntax ever so slightly and thus altered me completely. It was as though the lighting had been altered where a portrait was hung, thus changing the chiaroscuro completely and giving the subject much more depth.

As I observed the Minutemen whipping Georgetown through sheer determination, I understood that winning is a byproduct, not of physical ability, but of spiritual agility. The athletic prowess of great champions is not unlike the indomitable attitude of the British nation during World War II: Both are but manifestations of people's inner spirit.

As Ralph Waldo Emerson put this same proposition: "Self-trust is the essence of heroism."

Somehow, these small revelations about the winning spirit would begin to translate, over the coming months, into a new philosophy of active living and super-active management of my diabetes. I was becoming a new portrait of myself.

My Blood Sugar in All Its Guises

Another lesson learned during my bitter-sweet Provincetown vacation had to do with the physical exercise that has now become my main form of blood-sugar maintenance.

As a lifelong runner and habitual jock, exercise is what I do instinctively as a reaction to any crisis. Running has been my escape valve, my emotional balm, my psychotherapist, my spiritual advisor, my all-purpose alibi, my drug addiction, and my pain killer for more than 40 years now. My natural inclination, when I reached Provincetown licking my wounds in 1996, was to start running. In that context, I would go for long, soul-searching runs on the bike trails that snake through the sand dunes outside Provincetown.

It was beginning to dawn on me, as I padded through the ever-shifting sand dunes, that dealing with diabetes is a juggling act with many subtleties. The body of a diabetic is not unlike the fragile environment of this dunescape, where the geology, hydrology, wildlife, food chain, and human influences all interact in a delicate dance that determines the health of the whole system.

The dunes served as a metaphor for my own body. As someone with diabetes, I was now doomed to spend the rest of my life balancing a dizzying array of physical, psychological, and spiritual factors. My whole future depended on getting my diabetic ecology equalized within the shifting sand dunes of my bodily functions.

The key to this balancing trick, I was just beginning to comprehend, was my spiritual outlook, for that viewpoint would determine how effective I would be in handling my blood sugar and all its consequences.

Spirit, in effect, is the body's Gaea. Just as ecologists sometimes personify the planet as an earth mother, or Gaea, based on the metaphor of a Roman goddess, so the body can be defined by its own spirit, an earth mother generating the ecology of the whole bodily system.

Trapped in the Closet of My Own Body

As I ran through the dunelands, meditating on my newly diagnosed diabetes, I remembered an incident that had taken place some 20 years before in this same windswept place.

In the spring of 1976, I had been visiting a longtime friend of mine who now lived in Provincetown. One evening he suggested we bake some marijuana into a batch of Betty Crocker cookies. Having never had any appetite for either alcohol or drugs, I was much more interested in the cookies than the pot.

Late that night, after I had downed about a dozen Betty Crocker cookies, we sat lounging in my friend's cottage. For the past hour, we had been staring into a painting he had created, filled with scores of abstract images, both whimsical and haunting. Under the influence of the demon hemp, we were engaged in much the same activity as I would take up, years later, when confronted with Isabella Rossellini's portrait. We were deciphering all the hidden psychologies in the soul of the canvas.

That's when some kind of fearful genie was suddenly released by either my own mind or the drug itself. All at once, I realized that my body was a closet, and I was locked inside. Being an avid claustrophobic, I freaked out.

"I gotta get outta here!" I screamed, and ran out the door.

When I took off into the dunes outside P-town, my friend followed me. Fortunately, he was in exceedingly good condition, because at the time I was running about 70 hard miles per week. I must have run for four or five miles before I looked back to find him plugging along behind me.

That's when I sat down on one of the dunes and began rocking back and forth and crying.

"I'll never get away," is all I said, over and over.

I sat right there and rocked like that for the rest of the night, while my friend comforted me, as I tried to fathom what hidden symbols had been painted into the canvas of my soul.

Pentimento

Now, two decades later, I was running scared once more, this time from diabetes. I was suffering another mind-altering chemical crisis that had released another genie, which locked me in the closet of my body. And now it was going to take a period of adjustment before all my hormones, functions, and feelings reached a state of equilibrium.

As Lao-tzu, the founder of Taoism, once said, "Truth often sounds paradoxical." The paradoxical truth in this case was that facing myself was the only chance to escape from the closet of my own body.

By the end of my eventful week in Provincetown, I was beginning to understand the palette of change working at my spirit with its splashes of mystic paint. By no means did I have all the answers, nor even all the questions, about my diabetes. But I started to glimpse the reality of my situation and admit the brutal truth, which is the first step in any spiritual journey.

Being down and out in Provincetown was undoubtedly the blackest comedy I could ever invent for any vacation. And yet the experience had profound and long-lasting effects on my life. When God or Gaea or diabetes—Who knows which?—cursed me with this melancholy week, I was also given the greatest of all blessings in disguise: The beginnings of self-knowledge.

During that topsy-turvy week, I was also permanently fixed with the astrology of Cape Cod, as if influenced by a star configuration at my own rebirth. I would ever after be inspired by the gravitational pulls, the light waves, the tides, the stardust of the place.

Some mysterious element present in the mist, the fog, the shifting sands, and the positive ions of Cape Cod had turned it into my spiritual home, although I wouldn't know as much for quite some time. As you will see in the following pages, the permanent imprint of Cape Cod on my soul would become part and parcel of my five-year-long pilgrimage toward understanding, my own poor-man's version of enlightenment.

As Martha and I said good-bye to the Rossellini cottage, I remember turning at the bottom of the stairwell and glancing once more at the menacing portrait that had overseen the affairs of this week. At that moment the expression on this bastardized image of Isabella Rossellini appeared to have mellowed. It was as if the lines on her face had relaxed, the mouth had lost its digestive frown, the eyes had softened, the flesh had released the legion possessing it.

Who knows how such an optical illusion happens? Perhaps beauty is, indeed, in the eyes of the beholder. Then again, like a painting in progress, maybe each moment in life is merely tinged with, and reworked by, the innermost spirit of the person living it.

Or maybe I was experiencing a kind of pentimento, the phenomenon that occurs when old paint on canvas turns transparent. In the course of this pigmentary evanescence, the original lines, which were subsequently painted over as the artist altered the picture's image, sometimes come through the finished painting, changing it entirely. Maybe I was finally seeing pentimento taking place in the world around me, including Isabella's portrait, as the original lines came shining through the canvas I'd painted over with a lifetime of illusions.

I left the Cape with a newfound knowledge that was both profound and far-reaching. I was learning that one's own viewpoint can not only alter reality, but determine it. I was the painter of my own future.

At the same time, I was also sobered by all the hard work still left to be done. This realization was something like the letdown suffered after finding those fearsome words printed in small type on the packaging of so many modern-day devices:

"Some Assembly Required."

Now it was time for me to take my partially assembled new life and put it all together.

Okay, What Do I Do Now?

The Revolutionary Character of Diabetes

Almost two decades ago, my old friend, Tom Fix, sent me a postcard picturing his first-born child, Cora. On the back he had scribbled a brief message in the shaky handwriting of a new father.

"Okay, what do I do now?" he wrote.

That far-reaching question describes exactly how I felt throughout the spring of 1996, as I tried to understand the consequences of diabetes.

On the morning of June 15, Tom might well have been asking his astute question once again, as he and I went careening through the back streets of Amherst in my old Dodge pickup. Tom was beside himself because the butter-cream icing on my wedding cake, which he cradled in his lap, was melting all over his new Armani suit, one of the very few tokens of high fashion he'd ever purchased in his life.

I glanced at Tom while he was observing the runny confection staining his pants. The look on his face reminded me of the climactic scene from the 1951 film *The Thing (From Another World)*. This same horrific expression was glimpsed on the alien, played by James Arness, as he watched himself disintegrate from a powerful electric charge.

Our mission was to deliver the cake to the site of the reception, Seasons Restaurant, preferably before the dripping butter cream turned Tom into a large frosted ginger man. No doubt, at the moment, Tom was cursing the day he had ever agreed to fly cross-country from his home near Seattle and serve as my best man.

Fortunately, the cake was the only disaster on my wedding day. After Tom and I delivered the decomposing cake to Seasons, a team of culinary specialists went to work on my cake in an operation that must have resembled plastic surgery.

Tom was still wiping the icing off his only suit when we arrived at Smith College in nearby Northampton a half-hour later. Because Martha had graduated from Smith only days before as a non-traditional Ada Comstock Scholar, her new alumna status earned her the privilege of using the college's stately old chapel for her wedding.

It was an event blessed by loved ones from around the country and christened by the celestial sounds of Puccini arias and other heavenly music. We left the sound system in the hands of another old friend, Richard Farrell, who was stationed somewhere in the bowels of the chapel, operating the special effects like a latter-day Wizard of Oz. For his efforts during the ceremony, we began referring to Richard as the second best man.

Several special moments from our wedding day are especially pertinent to this story. One happened while Martha was being escorted up the aisle by her father as the angelic strains of Puccini's "Nessun Dorma" floated through the chapel, courtesy of the second best man.

I was spellbound by the sight of Martha in her lacy, old-fashioned wedding dress, her lovely and youthful face giving off an aura of ancient Bohemian beauty, passed down by her Czechoslovakian ancestors. In Jungian fashion, her archetypal image brought all the emotional turbulence of the past few months to the surface.

Not only was I overwhelmed by the elegance and decency of the woman who was about to take my hand in marriage, but also by the roller coaster of dealing with diabetes. In this sense, I was still adjusting to the minute by minute emotions of having diabetes: feeling my mood swing whenever my blood sugar took a plunge; wondering how diabetes might shorten my life span; fearing the terrible complications; experiencing the constant emotional pressure of daily management. These uneasy sensations were giving my life the stability of an amusement park ride. And now I let loose.

All this emotion turned me into a blubbering idiot.

Our ring-bearer was a full-blooded collie named Louis, often referred to as "the Buddha dog" by his owners, our dear old friends, Terry Allen and Ernie Urvater. When Louis came ambling down the aisle with the ring attached to his collar, everyone else in the chapel howled with laughter. Everyone but me, that is. I was still sobbing uncontrollably.

Later, at the reception, a local band named Salamander Crossing was playing bluegrass and country swing, but nobody was dancing. This was staid old Massachusetts, after all. At one point, Martha, who is normally the most mild-mannered and soft-spoken of people, pointed at several tables filled with friends and colleagues.

"You!" she said with the voice of unquestioned authority. "I want you out on that dance floor right now!"

The response was instantaneous. Like raw recruits obeying their drill sergeant, people from all over the restaurant jerked to their feet and flooded toward the dance floor.

Later, I pulled Martha aside.

"What got into you?" I said with some awe and no little admiration.

Martha regarded me with that sly smile she gets when discovering anything new about herself.

"It's just that, with my wedding dress on," she said, "I sense this unlimited power."

For all intents and purposes, Martha in her wedding dress was functioning with all the authority of an apparition by the Blessed Virgin Mary.

Why does this incident still tickle me every time I think about it? Because here was yet more proof that human beings possess unleashed potential—"this unlimited power," as Martha phrased it—for changing reality and controlling their own destiny.

"If you would be a complete person," said 19th-century Puerto Rican activist Eugenio Maria de Hostos, "put all your soul's strength into all your life's actions."

A Stranger in a Strange Land

As for me, I was putting all my soul's strength into diabetes.

By the time of the wedding, my new condition had denatured my very being. Anyone who has ever been mutated by the insidious fallout of this disease knows at once what I mean. I was a stranger entering a strange new land.

To begin with, I had revamped my whole work life at UMass as I adjusted to my blood sugar and the oral medication I was taking. Everything I did on campus was dictated by diabetes: from making sure I had a bite to eat before any big meeting, so I could avoid low-blood-sugar attacks, to taking regular meditation breaks, so I could moderate stress.

As part of this new lifestyle, I kept my glucose-monitoring kit on my office desk so I could test myself throughout the day. Of course, it also took me five minutes of heavy-duty pushups and jumping jacks before I could get my blood pumping well enough to squeeze a drop on each test strip. Sometimes colleagues would walk into my office and catch me at these peculiar pursuits, which must have added to my reputation as an odd duck.

As part of my new ritual, I always visited the snack bar for take-out food after my first glucose reading of the morning. Through trial and error, I arrived at the best item on the menu to help me tiptoe across that tightrope between hypoglycemia and hyperglycemia that every person with diabetes walks. My comfort food, in this case, was a grilled bagel I took back to my office and seasoned with artificial sweetener and cinnamon; a curious concoction, for sure, but one that satisfied my sweet tooth while keeping my blood sugar in check.

Once, while I was fixing a bagel at my desk, a co-worker popped in for a visit. My visitor was not a very close friend. In fact, he didn't even know I had diabetes. But we had become chummy over the years, despite his annoying habit of blurting out tactless remarks. In that respect, I often referred to him as Mr. Freudian Slip.

When he saw me sprinkling packets of artificial sweetener on my bagel, Mr. Freudian Slip smirked.

"What are you doing to that bagel?" he said. "Where I come from, that's called a sacrilege."

This harmless remark must have caught me in a moment of weakness, because it really pissed me off. I had to muster every ounce of self-control to hold my tongue.

"Wherever you come from," I thought, "why don't you crawl back in your hole?"

Why was I so steamed? Maybe because that little bagel had come to symbolize the total nutritional reform I'd been forced to make in my diet. My morning bagel represented the Diabetic Paradox: you need enough nutrition to stop from dipping into low blood sugar, but, at the same time, you must avoid any food or any amount of it that might send your blood sugar skyrocketing.

That same paradox became all too apparent, and all too dangerous, when I was exercising. This lesson was driven home within a week after I went on oral medication, during one of my initial five-mile runs under the new regime of Glynase. After a couple of miles, I experienced my first bout with low-blood sugar. A feeling of overwhelming weakness came over me, accompanied by disorientation, confusion, shaking limbs, and a roaring urge for sweetness.

Fortunately, I wasn't far from my house and was able to stagger home and guzzle a jumbo glass of orange juice. But if I had chosen a more far-flung running route that day, I might be dead right now.

Soon thereafter, I consulted a professor in the Exercise Science Department at UMass who advised me to take an energy bar with me whenever I ran or played any other sport.

"But won't that be bad for my blood sugar?" I said.

"On the contrary," she told me. "It could save your life and stop you from going into coma."

Reshaping Me in Fundamental Ways

Meanwhile, diabetes was reshaping my outlook in many fundamental ways, both large and small. First of all, it refocused my whole viewpoint on work. Before diabetes, I regarded my job at UMass as a necessary evil. "Work is anything anybody else wants you do to," as my second best man, Richard Farrell, had once observed. Still, I needed that gig to make a living, pay the mortgage, and support the poetry and fiction that are my passions as a writer.

But looking at life through the fisheye lens of diabetes, I now viewed the hours I spent at UMass— almost a third of my life—as a monumental waste of time. Diabetes had convinced me that the sands were quickly running out in my hourglass. I didn't want to squander what little time I had left by writing PR puff pieces that nobody really needed.

I soon developed what most supervisors would call a "bad attitude," based on the simple fact I didn't want to be there. The symptoms were cynicism, boredom, and wisecracks, which would often jump out of my mouth at staff meetings.

With this altered consciousness came a restless bodily sensation, which would take over my system as I was working at my computer on one meaningless project or another. It was as if an ant colony were using my arteries as its nest. I could actually feel the little devils streaming through me. At first, I thought this disturbing phenomenon might be some physical effect of diabetes, but it wasn't. Gradually, I realized the ants were my own emotions, telling me I was frittering away my life.

Aside from this impatient new outlook, I bridled at the cumulative effect from scores of minor incidents that happened every week. A short list of these

"Diabetic Moments," as I call them, should sound all too familiar to most readers:

- each time a wait person offered me a dessert menu
- every time a friend asked if I'd like a cocktail
- whenever a colleague brought donuts to an office meeting
- each time a newscaster announced the death of another celebrity who had passed away due to "complications from diabetes"
- any of numerous social situations when propriety forced me to answer the kindness of strangers by saying, "No, thank you, I have diabetes"
- whenever I read another newspaper article about the "diabetes epidemic" in America
- each time I saw someone with an amputated limb
- anything that reminded me about the crippling effects of stroke, neuropathy, kidney disease, or retinal failure

Each of these events might have caused only one minor ripple in my psyche, but all of them put together amounted to a wave of terror. I was reminded of an old movie I'd seen many years before, one called *The Naked Jungle*, in which a huge swarm of insatiable red ants went rampaging through a South American forest, devouring all the soft vegetation in its path. What the ants left behind was the skeleton of a jungle.

That image, in fact, was what diabetes was doing to my emotions, leaving them naked, frayed, and exposed.

Lasting Impressions

Even seemingly incidental conversations began leaving lasting impressions. For example, one of my best friends once had a serious bout with cancer that she survived in a very heroic way. I wasn't even thinking about her own medical history the day I broke the news I had diabetes.

"It's got me a little psyched out," I told her, hoping for a word of solace.

She stared into the distance for a moment.

"I know how you feel," she finally said. "Though it could be a lot worse."

I knew precisely what she meant. This episode served as a healthy slap in the face and a permanent cure for my self-pity.

One of the most telling events of this kind happened when a type 1 friend suffered a dangerous low-blood-sugar incident at a restaurant. We had just ordered and were chatting about something pleasant, when Rick, as I'll call him here, began too look a little dazed and confused. Then he started repeating the same phrase over and over again.

"Are you in trouble, buddy?" I said.

When he nodded, I ran to the bartender and told him my friend was having a hypoglycemic attack. By the time I got back to our table with a glass of orange juice, Rick was shaking uncontrollably. He was in such a state, he couldn't even swallow. It was apparent he was losing consciousness.

"Just relax," I told Rick as he bent over the juice trying to make his straw work, "and take one good sip at a time."

I held the glass for him and kept talking.

"That's right," I said. "Now rest for a second and then try again."

The situation was touch and go for the next ten minutes. Despite spilling orange juice all over his work clothes, Rick kept sipping. I could see he was focusing all his concentration and will power into the simple act of coaxing juice through that little straw.

Later, he would tell me his blood-sugar reading must have dipped to 20.

After Rick had recovered somewhat, I said, "Man, you'd do anything to keep me entertained at lunch."

All my joking aside, I probably felt even more shaken than he did. After all, I had just seen the day-to-day struggle of every person with diabetes embodied in his predicament. As much as we each try to lead a normal life untouched by our condition, it can all break down at any moment.

"There but for fortune," as the classic Joan Baez song expressed this truism, "go you and I."

Nothing Lost on Martha

As many people with diabetes discover, chronic illness is often more difficult on one's spouse than oneself. The dangers of diabetes were never lost on Martha. Indeed, the symptoms of the disease broke out in our relationship more frequently than in my own organism.

As just one example, my entire diet soon underwent a total transformation: from fewer red meats, carbohydrates, and fatty foods to more vegetables, whole grains, fresh fruit, and fish. Because of my needs, Martha willingly changed her eating habits as well. Before long, our menu bore little resemblance to the rich foods we had enjoyed in the past. But, as always, Martha brushed away any allusions to her own self-sacrifice.

"No use both of us going monastic," I once told her.

"Our new diet is healthier for both of us," she said.

Our changing diet also disturbed the courting rituals that make any love affair special. For instance, sharing ice cream, pastry, or gooey confections had always been our most hallowed romantic rite. Now, except for special occasions, we both chose to forego our just desserts.

Nobody should ever underestimate the conflict of a sugarman or sugarwoman with a real sweet tooth, nor the sacrifices of a spouse trying to help.

As with any serious disease, diabetes preyed on our relationship in many surreptitious ways. For example, Martha understood all too well the risks of diabetes. She not only worried about the many ways that diabetes can manifest itself in long-term complications, but also the danger from acute low-blood-sugar attacks. I wish I had a nickel for every time

she's asked, "Do you have a sweet with you?" when
I went off to exercise.

The subtle stresses of diabetes would sometimes
flare up without any warning. Martha and I seldom
argue and almost never raise our voices to each other. In
fact, we regard our civility toward one another as both
a strength and a weakness. Though there are many
rewards to the practice of tolerance, it doesn't allow the
escape valve of a good old knock-down, drag-out fight.

One exception to our good-natured relationship
took place several months after I was diagnosed with
diabetes. My knowledge was still sketchy about the
disease, and my fears about such complications as skin
infections were operating on what the government
would call "a heightened state of alert." As I would
soon prove, there's a fine line between alertness and
paranoia.

As it happened, Martha and I were in the process
of moving, and at the time I was mopping the living
room floor in the house we were leaving. That's when I
accidentally jammed a large splinter into my stocking
foot. At this point, I pitched a fit.

When Martha tried to calm me down, I screamed,
"Don't you get it? Something like this could kill me!"

"What I don't get," she said, "is why you're
yelling like that. What I don't get is why you're taking
it out on me."

She was right, of course. Besides apologizing, I
had to take a hard look at what diabetes was doing to
me, and what, in turn, I was doing to my friends and
loved ones. I didn't want to spend the rest of my life
taking out my frustrations on innocent bystanders,

such as Martha with the splinter, or Mr. Freudian Slip with the bagel.

I had to ask, "What must I change to be happy with diabetes?" The answer was my whole frame of reference. But I wouldn't realize for some time that such far-reaching change is more an act of spiritual revolution than an act of will. Your worldview can never be transformed unless your soul is deeply touched first.

This truth, in fact, would ultimately become the theme of my whole future as a person dealing with diabetes.

Finding Myself Embedded in All That Marble

My Search for the Inner Sugarman

"Once you've spewed out a first draft," wrote author Anne Lamott, "the worst is over and then you can go back. It is like Michelangelo finding the statue of David in all that marble."

Likewise, once I had been diagnosed with diabetes and gone through an initial period of trials and tribulations, the first draft of my new life had been completed. The worst was over. Now all I had to do was find myself embedded in all that marble. My inner search would take the next five years and counting.

In the months following my wedding, the overpowering emotions brought on by diabetes were beginning to subside, gradually replaced by a vague feeling of uneasiness. This was the precursor of the spiritual revolution I was about to undergo.

South African writer Nadine Gordimer once described the slow process I was going through over this span of time: "It is not the conscious changes made in their lives by men and women—a new job, a new town, a divorce—which really shape them, like the chapter headings in a biography, but a long slow mutation of emotion, hidden, all-penetrative. . . ."

Certainly I was mutating in an all-penetrating way. But what was I becoming?

The Great Snipe Hunt

As I said above, I was quickly growing disillusioned with my monotonous duties as Senior Writer at UMass, where I had little work, and too much time to do it.

On a daily basis, as I stared out my window in the hermetically sealed environment of the main administration building, I started to realize that the symptoms of my own dissatisfaction are part of an epidemic in this country. A burgeoning population suffers from a common complex of indications that include:

- a free-floating sense of meaninglessness
- the fear that our life's work is of no redeeming social value
- the urge to do something dramatic without having the slightest idea what it might be
- a notion that something quite essential is missing in our lifestyle

- an overarching feeling of boredom, despite being bombarded with media stimuli during every waking hour
- a powerful impulse to flee

The end result of this widespread disillusion is a land rife with the alienation described by Henry David Thoreau in *Walden*: "The mass of people lead lives of quiet desperation."

I once spotted a group of Russian Orthodox monks, dressed in their traditional black robes and wearing their customary long beards, gathered around an automated teller, arguing loudly as they tried to figure out how to make the money come out. To me that scene has always embodied a world in which tradition, civility, and culture have been displaced by future shock.

American writer Susan Sontag blames much of our disillusion on the "inhuman acceleration of historical change." She calls the resulting alienation "intellectual vertigo."

To me, as a 50-year-old person with diabetes who was undergoing intellectual vertigo, existence seemed like one huge "Snipe Hunt," that clever trick played on new campers as a type of hazing when I was a Boy Scout in 1956.

The modus operandi of a Snipe Hunt was to wake all the young Tenderfoots in the wee hours of the morning and send them reeling into the dark chasing after imaginary snipes (which in the real world are inland sandpipers similar to woodcocks. But this wasn't the real world). The illusion of the hunt was carried out by older scouts, who were hiding in the bushes making snipe calls and imitating the sounds of birds thrashing through the underbrush.

I remember my first Snipe Hunt, at Grapevine Lake near Dallas. After chasing phantom snipes for what seemed like an eternity, I found myself tired, sweaty, confused, and lost in a dark thicket. All around me, I could hear the sounds of chaos, as "snipes" shrieked, Tenderfoots howled, and flashlight beams spider-webbed the woods. "Who cares?" I finally said to myself, and sat down right where I was to wait for daybreak. I suppose that attitude is why I never advanced past Tenderfoot.

Now, four decades later, I was still a Tenderfoot chasing a subspecies of snipes: the illusive spiritual principles that give life meaning. Even though I could still hear the snipes calling, and I could still make out their thrashing in the woods, I never seemed to catch one.

But at least I was gradually coming to understand the nature of the Great Snipe Hunt we are all on. During the months following my wedding, as I regarded life through the new eyes of a person with diabetes, I began to catch fleeting glimpses of the snipes that many of us, from many walks of life, are chasing so futilely.

Fluttering Right into My Waiting Hands

During the last few months of 1996, I stepped up my search for snipes by scanning the stacks of local bookstores in Amherst for titles that offered some glimmer of hope for my future.

Strangely enough, a few publications seemed to jump off the shelves like flushed birds. Suddenly, after all these years of snipe hunting, the illusory prey was coming to life and fluttering right into my waiting hands. Over the next few years, I would read a succession of books that significantly altered my outlook on life.

The first book that flew into my fingers was *Care of the Soul: A Guide for Cultivating Depth and Sacredness in Everyday Life* by Thomas Moore, a well-known archetypal psychologist and lecturer. What might have attracted me to this work was the notation on the back cover that Moore had lived as a Catholic monk for 12 years. I've had a fondness for monasteries ever since my own time as an accidental monk. Monasticism had become one of my favorite archetypal images.

For me, Moore got right to the quick of the spiritual crisis in our culture. "The great malady of the twentieth century, implicated in all our troubles and affecting us individually and socially," he wrote in his introduction, "is 'loss of soul.'"

He listed several common maladies of the soul that therapists hear everyday in their practices.

- emptiness
- meaninglessness
- vague depression
- disillusionment about marriage, family, and relationships
- loss of values

- yearning for personal fulfillment
- a hunger for spirituality

Each complaint indicates loss of soul, and I could relate to every one. Unlike many therapists, Moore's answer to all this quiet desperation was not years of psychoanalysis or, worse still, a flood of psychobabble. His resolution was creating depth in one's soul by carrying on a daily practice of spirituality, much as a monk might do. His eloquent wisdom and observations about how to do so still serve as continuing inspiration for me today.

My next discovery was an oldie but goodie: *The Art of Loving* by renowned psychoanalyst Erich Fromm. What boggled me about this classic work was his simple but brilliant deduction about the source of all human anxiety. It is created by loneliness. In his book, Fromm's far-reaching definition of the human being was "life being aware of itself." But the human gift for self-awareness is both a blessing and a curse, because through it each person realizes that he or she is a separate, lonely entity. How? We each know about our short life span. We each understand how we were born and will perish without any say in our destiny. We each comprehend that we will either die before our loved ones, or they will die before us. We each realize our own helplessness before the overwhelming forces of nature and society.

"All this," Fromm deduced, "makes each person's separate, disunited existence an unbearable prison."

Fromm's solution to our separateness was a powerful formula, detailed in his book, for practicing *The Art of Loving*.

Another book that enriched my hunt for
knowledge was *The Art of Happiness*, a collaborative
book authored by Howard C. Cutler, M.D., based on
his discussions with His Holiness the Dalai Lama.

"I believe that the very purpose of our life is to
seek happiness," said the Dalai Lama. "That is clear.
Whether one believes in religion or not, whether one
believes in this religion or that religion, we are all
seeking something better in life. So, I think, the very
motion of our life is towards happiness."

The problem, as the Dalai Lama concluded in
The Art of Happiness, is that happiness is not a state of
bliss, like the Garden of Eden, that we simply inherit
and inhabit as our birth rite. Rather, it is the end
result of a very disciplined and structured way of
thinking, which takes many years to develop, and a
lifetime to perfect.

"Permanent happiness can only be achieved,"
said the Dalai Lama, "through training the mind."

In that respect, happiness is an art form, and like
all forms of art, it can only be perfected by perseverance,
hard work, discipline, and the employment of our innate
gifts, a process explored in depth by *The Art of Happiness*.

The next book I bought was *Awakening to the
Sacred: Creating a Spiritual Life from Scratch* by Lama
Surya Das. He's an American-born author who has
spent 30 years studying Buddhism with the great
masters of Asia, including the Dalai Lama. I probably
bought this volume because of its very first line. "If you
have picked up this book, then in all probability you
are a seeker." Yes, I thought. Not only a seeker, but
a snipe hunter.

What I liked about the approach of Lama Surya Das was that he integrated Buddhist thought with many other spiritual philosophies and traditions, while showing readers how to create personalized spiritual practices based on their own beliefs, outlooks, goals, and needs. As you can tell from contrasting the title and subtitle, the author also combined the Eastern gift for elevated wisdom with the Western penchant for down-to-earth lingo.

Before long, I was using a large number of insightful suggestions from this book to begin whipping up my own homemade spiritual life, totally from scratch.

One more book that had a great effect on me as I tried to locate the snipes in my life was *The Best Spiritual Writing of 1998*, edited by Smith College professor Philip Zaleski. In his preface, Zaleski told an amusing tale about strolling down the main street of a small New England town with his friend, a Benedictine Monk, who was dressed in monastic robes. Usually, such an outfit would have gone unnoticed, but today the monk's garb was attracting a lot of attention. "Looking good!" shouted a tattooed biker sitting at a sidewalk café. "Wild outfit," commented a teenage girl. Not until they finished their walk did the two friends realize it was Halloween. Everyone on the sidewalk had assumed the monk was in costume.

The story serves as a good metaphor for the new way that many unlikely people are beginning to look at spiritual practices, such as monasticism. To that biker and teenager, the monk's costume must have seemed exotic, creative, humorous, and even romantic.

Likewise, many other people, such as myself, are seeing spirituality with new eyes.

In this book, I found soulful essays by a diverse assortment of people viewing spirituality from many angles. This book reinforced in my mind that spirituality encompasses a range of human experiences not traditionally regarded as spiritual. For many people, running and other sports are blessed events that exercise the soul as well as the body. For others, they discover their innermost selves while hiking or birdwatching or camping or communing with nature. Simple silence is a spiritual act for many soul-seekers. Even the act of struggle is a spiritual process: striving for perfection; striving to create art; striving to make oneself into a better person; striving to exhibit a can-do attitude; striving, as people with diabetes must, to control chronic illness. All these states are spiritual in nature. Potentially, we are all monastics, practicing our faith with our own personalized creeds, dressed in the robes of our own individual spirits.

"There is no end," said Patricia Hampl in her introduction to *The Best Spiritual Writing of 1998*, "to the human habit of finding meaning."

The Best Spiritual Writing of 1998 was a key document in my own spiritual development because, for the first time, it gave me the inspiration to write about my own spiritual issues.

During the next few years of reading and seeking, I was influenced by many other books. I looked into the synthesized philosophy of Deepak Chopra. I delved into the mystical world of Alan Watts. I entertained Steve Hagen's plain and simple explanation of Buddhism. I wrestled with David Rosen's interpretation of Carl Jung as a kind of Taoist. I considered the basics of yoga as explained by Godfrey Devereaux. I enjoyed spiritually based novels by Barbara Kingsolver, Anne Tyler, and Graham Greene. I devoured the poetry of Gary Snyder, Pablo Neruda, Walt Whitman, García Lorca, and Charles Simic.

All this writing inspired me to develop a number of spiritual practices, centered around meditation and reading and other healing habits that I believed would provide a lifelong structure for my metaphysical questing. I detail this systematic approach to soulful living in part 3 of *Zen and the Art of Diabetes Maintenance*.

A Monument to Nonentity

Meanwhile, the spirituality found in the works I was reading also left me with several unresolved issues. For one thing, nothing in any of the bookstores spoke to the special spiritual needs of a person with diabetes.

"How do I find the inspiration," I kept asking myself, "for dealing with the daily grind of controlling my blood sugar?"

Another related matter concerned the nature of my livelihood: how to put my fledgling spirituality to work in my career and make my employment meaningful to myself and others.

One thing you need to understand about my job was that the administrator who hired me in 1993 had been fired several months later, I trust through no fault

of my own. Since then I had been passed like a
counterfeit bill from supervisor to supervisor, six of
them in all, none of whom had the slightest idea what
I was supposed to be doing. The actual concept for my
original position had long ago been lost in the dustbin
of institutional memory.

Every day at UMass I was becoming more of a
persona non grata, at least in my own eyes. My position
was a monument to nonentity.

Into the Haunted House
One at a Time

My philosophical snipe-hunting caused me to
evolve quite slowly in an all-penetrating way, a
mutation that went on for much of the next three
years.

One cardinal rule of a good story is to create
competent and effective characters. Nothing is more
irritating than watching a movie in which the
characters can't seem to grasp the obvious. You might
call this the "Let's Send Each Teenager into the
Haunted House One at a Time to Die" approach
to story-telling.

The problem with real life is that too many of us
are incompetent characters wearing blinders. That's
why it took me several years of denial before I would
accept the idea conking me on the noggin, the naked
truth about what I should do with my life.

Then one day in early1999 I was sitting in a staff
meeting with my colleagues from the communications

office, some of whom I'd known for 20 years. Understandably, I had developed a great fondness for most of these people.

As the boring agenda droned on, I glanced from one face to the next. I knew for a fact that none of my associates was happy. Nobody wanted to be here, now or ever. Most of us were lifers, working in jobs we didn't believe in, merely because the pay was decent, the benefits gave us a sense of security, and the state annuity plan would support us in our old age. I suspect we all knew, down to the last minute, when we were each eligible to collect our own pensions.

Like the myopic protagonists in numerous drive-in schlock flicks, each of us was being sent into the haunted house one at a time to die.

"Is this what life is all about?" I asked myself as I sat there in that meeting. "A job whose only ultimate purpose is the retirement package?"

"Charlie," my current supervisor noted during a lull in the conversation. "You look like you've got a lot on your mind."

"You don't want to hear it," I said.

No Offense Shall Go Un-imagined

That meeting might not have given me the inspiration I needed to change my life, but it certainly served as a key part of the process.

I love UMass, which is my alma mater, after all, and has provided a fine education for thousands of productive citizens. It's definitely the most underrated education in New England. But I was finding it harder and harder to go to work each day, not because I didn't believe in the institution, but because of the general negativity in my department. Any workplace filled with so many longtime employees seems to grow a bacterial culture all its own, one blooming with competitiveness, jealousy, backbiting, gossip, and power plays.

In that respect, UMass rivaled the Roman Empire in terms of political intrigue.

As just one example from hundreds, I once proposed to work on a new interactive Web site that would have solved numerous communications problems. My motive for this suggestion was total boredom, since a Hack Writer in Residence has so little actual work to do. Within minutes of my proposal being made public, two of my colleagues went banging on our supervisor's office door to complain about my expansionist policies. Evidently, no territory of such size had been threatened since Germany invaded the Soviet Union during World War II.

This incident proved once again the basic law governing any hard-core bureaucracy:

"No offense shall go un-imagined."

I eventually got this message and stopped looking for work to do. One day, as I was sequestered in my office pretending I had duties to perform, I read a passage from *Awakening the Buddha Within*, yet another elegant book by Lama Surya Das. This excerpt might not have awakened the Buddha within, but it certainly aroused the sleeping giant that was my potential.

In this chapter, the author advised me as the reader to ask myself the following challenging questions about my job:

> Is my work life mostly composed of chores and compromises, responsibilities, duties, and obligations? Or am I passionately engaged in following my own star? What would I do differently if I could?. . . Is my field of endeavor basically honest, meaningful, and helpful to myself and others . . .? Is it emotionally fulfilling: financially, psychologically, and socially rewarding; engaging, creatively satisfying, and bringing the best out of me through utilizing and further developing my own unique combinations of special gifts, talents, experiences, and interests? Does my work . . . contribute to a brighter, happier, safer world and a better society? Is there anything I am putting off until later that might best be undertaken now?. . .What is keeping me from doing that?

After reading this passage from *Awakening the Buddha Within* and thinking it over for several days, something indeed stirred within my consciousness. I realized my job was woefully inadequate in almost every important aspect. The only thing my work provided was security, which in some ways is the worst jinx of all. How many friends did I have who were being suffocated by their own security?

The Momentum of Everyday Habits

In many ways, momentum is the most difficult of all addictions to change. Many of the unhappiest people I know are maintained solely by the momentum of their everyday habits. They are the J. Alfred Prufrocks of this world, who, like T.S. Elliot's timid protagonist, measure out their lives with coffee spoons.

One of those was me.

Then one workaday morning, as I was staring blankly at one of my speeches, full of sound and fury and indicating nothing on my computer screen, the idea hit me; not as a blinding flash of enlightenment, mind you, but as more of an afterthought. Why didn't I think of this before?

No one, to my knowledge, had ever written the kind of spiritual guide for people with diabetes that I so desperately needed for my own benefit. I was a writer. I was also a person with diabetes trying to understand the spiritual nature of existence. Perhaps there were more lost souls like me.

So, why didn't I just write the book myself?

In Eastern philosophy, such an idea involves that part of dharma, or the natural moral law of the universe, which relates to performing "right conduct" in your livelihood. One basic concept of right conduct in your work is to take what you've learned and create something of value for other people.

"The superior person understands what is right," as Confucius explained the basic tenet of any meaningful livelihood. "The inferior person understands what will sell."

During the next few months, as I organized my thoughts about *Zen and the Art of Diabetes Maintenance* and began putting them into a book proposal, the project gave me a sense of purpose and direction that I had rarely experienced before.

The inspiration I received from doing the right thing also had immediate physical effects on my diabetes. The very act of putting my beliefs into action, while simultaneously carrying out a daily routine of spiritual practices, inspired me to live my life more fully and manage my blood sugar better.

Inspiration was now infusing my life and all its issues. What's more, as I ruefully noted to myself, this inspiration was also the end result of the sugar that had once infused my body and all its tissues.

New Beginnings, Further Consequences

"Every beginning is a consequence," wrote French poet Paul Valéry.

If every beginning is a consequence, each consequence in turn triggers new beginnings and further consequences. This continuum forms the great cycle of human development and the chain reaction of spiritual seeking.

Thus, as I worked on *Zen and the Art of Diabetes Maintenance*, I was also coming to some troubling conclusions about my life that would soon set off a domino effect. It was dawning on me that, for me to complete the journey I was starting with this book, I had to make several key life changes as well. After all, any pilgrimage worth taking at all means giving up a few comforts along the way.

I sensed something essentially wrong with my easy lifestyle in the pretty landscape of western Massachusetts, known fittingly as "Happy Valley." Fortunately for me, Martha was reaching the same conclusions I was, and precisely at the same time. Or maybe here was yet one more demonstration of the synchronicity that links all being.

We both intuited something fundamentally unrewarding about our jobs, our suburban way of life, and the mortgage it was all supporting. As actor Anthony Quinn, in his defining role as Zorba the Greek, summed up this vicious cycle of work, lifestyle, and home-ownership:

"Yes, I had it all. A house, family, a job. The whole catastrophe!"

Martha and I spent many a dinnertime talking about the disenchantment that was welling up in our lives. We were living the American Dream and hated it.

One day, sometime in the winter of 1999, Martha and I sat down in the kitchen of our heavily mortgaged little farmhouse and began listing what was missing from our lives, what we wanted instead, and where we might go to get it. Although our list filled several sheets of paper, we never did reach a bottom line about an ultimate "destination," in any sense of that word; maybe because, as every story-teller knows, the most satisfying ending is also the hardest to see coming. Nevertheless, after many weeks of fretting and conversing, we finally figured out how to begin our journey toward understanding. With the first step.

That's how we came to the conclusion that would bring about the final stage of my metamorphosis, as triggered by diabetes three years before. Martha and I decided on the hardest path either of us had ever taken. We would quit our jobs, sell our house, and begin a pilgrimage to find our spiritual home, wherever that might lead us.

"Buddha did the same thing," as I explained our logic to one skeptical crony of mine. "He quit his plush life in the palace of his father and became a wandering nomad. With my screwed-up past, I need it a hell of a lot more than he did."

When our friends found out about our bizarre course of action, they were understandably horrified. They called it the worst kind of mid-life crisis. One buddy blamed my decision on a bad case of "precocious senility." My extended family, which had seen my flights of fancy before, no doubt chalked it all up to my highly cultivated immaturity.

Meanwhile, at work I was regarded as the Candide of the central administration, a naive fool in search of an impossible ideal. I remember one conversation I had with a pal of mine who was patiently biding his time until his handsome retirement plan kicked-in.

"Now, let me get this straight," he said after I informed him of our scheme. "You're going to quit your job because it's too easy and you don't have enough work?"

"That's about the gist of it," I said.

"And you're going to sell your house because it's too nice and cozy?"

"Yep."

"And you're going to leave Happy Valley because it's too comfortable?"

"Right."

"And then what?"

"We're liquidating our assets so we can go on a spiritual quest."

My friend nodded sagely as he considered the totality of this information.

"Tell me again," he finally said. "Why are you doing all this?"

Don't Hear the Bell, Be the Bell

Embarking on a Spiritual Pilgrimage

On Friday the 13th in August, 1999,
Martha and I signed the closing papers on
our little farmhouse, locked all our belongings in three
storage units across the street from the UMass football
stadium, and rode off into the western sunset bound for
destinations unknown.

"You cannot travel the path," the Buddha once
said, "before you have become the Path itself."

For the first time in a life full of travel and
adventure and relocation, I had become the Path itself,
a search for self-knowledge manifested in the very
journey I was taking. Yes, I was quitting yet one more
job and leaving yet one more place, as I'd done so many
times in my earlier years. But now, after all that
running away from reality, I was finally running toward

it. Instead of fooling myself, as I'd done so often during my quixotic search for adventure, love, fame, and fortune, now, at last, I was chasing my innermost spirit, wherever that might lead me.

At least, that's what I kept telling myself. Time and tide would tell if I was right or not.

We spent the next six months looking for something that might not exist—a spiritual dwelling place—in hopes that its very nonexistence might bring it to life. If this sounds like an impossible dream, it wasn't. In the end our trip accomplished exactly what we had envisioned. It's just that the pilgrimage didn't happen exactly the same way it did in our vision.

After visiting with the remnants of my family, living along the Front Range of the Colorado Rockies, Martha and I signed on as seasonal hospitality workers on the South Rim of the Grand Canyon.

The Big Ditch, as the local staff often called the canyon, certainly seemed like a logical place to start our pilgrimage, for in many ways this geologic masterpiece is considered the symbolic soul of the continent. Not only is it the most renowned of the world's Seven Wonders, but the Grand Canyon occupies a hallowed place in the history of the national parks, the spirit of the West, and the consciousness of the nation. People come from every nation to stare into this immense formation and bask in its spirit. Few geologic formations outside of the Himalayas and the oceans hold so much human symbolism. It's one of America's archetypal images.

I hired on as a porter in Grand Canyon Village, where I worked in the Bright Angel Lodge, El Tovar

Hotel, and other facilities. My job was to clean the public lounges and rest rooms, and to transport extra pillows, portable beds, toiletries, and other items to the guest rooms. I considered myself the world's oldest errand boy.

To celebrate my new job, I sent postcards to friends describing myself in my porter's uniform douching out urinals. "This might be the only job," I wrote, "that my English degree and 25 years of writing experience really qualify me to do."

Martha's position was somewhat more dignified, but also a good deal more irritating, than mine. She worked the front desk at the Bright Angel Lodge and, as such, had to field a battery of stupid questions and petty complaints every day; things like "Why do the sunrise bus tours all leave so early?" and "Why isn't the canyon lit up all night so we can see it?"

Our jobs didn't have many fringe benefits, but the one advantage was working on the brink of this natural phenomenon, the Grand Canyon. While emptying the garbage cans along the rim, which was another one of my solemn duties as porter, there was always time to stand for a while and gaze into the air-brushed depths of the world's most famous wonder.

Out there the cliffs fell away, as far as the eye could see, into yawning shapes of every color and texture. It was like communicating with deities.

The air in this immense crevasse seemed to shine, seemed to emit its own inner glory, so clear and far-reaching and beatific, magnifying infinity and defying time. The rosy clarity of the atmosphere made it possible to pick out details of rock formations many miles away. Each moment seemed to hang suspended in space, the way the great condors did, those endangered birds, thriving here after being transplanted from California.

I had never seen anything like the sedimented colors in the walls of the canyon, the ribbons of tawny yellow and cinnabar and rust-stone and salamander and carmine and luster-leaf and carnation and fossil-resin, all seeming to resonate. They were so still, and yet in their stillness they harbored the eternal motion of the universe. The atoms and molecules might have been conspiring to make the inanimate live. The canyon held all the stability of stone and all the fluidity of seawater in its dance of fortitude and flux.

In many ways, it was the same as gazing into one's own soul.

Drug Addicts, Deranged Criminals, and Other Colorful Employees

Unfortunately, our employment with the corporation that ran the Grand Canyon concessions didn't leave us much off-time to enjoy the canyon, and the company's personnel-screening methods left something to be desired. As Groucho Marx might have said, "Why would I want to work anywhere that would hire me?"

For reasons better left unexplained, the hospitality industry at the Grand Canyon attracted a large percentage of tough guys, dysfunctional alcoholics, lost souls, drug addicts, deranged criminals, and other employees of every stripe.

Strange as it might seem, I liked many of the castaways in this eccentric cast of players. One friend's passion was visiting the gravesites of every famous outlaw and hoodlum in American history. His current goal was a pilgrimage to the burial plots of Bonnie and Clyde. Another of my pals was gently obsessed with high school football and traveled hundreds of miles on his off days searching out the best games in the West. One guy on my crew was a Navajo Indian, paradoxically named Cowboy, who spent many of his vacations on vision quests and other Native American rites. Yet another fellow porter was a former member of a Los Angeles street gang.

I learned to respect and admire all these people. Unfortunately, there was also a large number of sinister jokers who gave the whole culture a dangerous feel to it and, in the end, poisoned the atmosphere of the village. There were often loud arguments and drunken brawls in the dormitories, alarming fights that kept Martha and me awake all night and ruined our mood for days to come.

Many of these outbreaks occurred on Wednesday night, which was no coincidence, since Wednesday was payday. By Thursday, many of the paychecks were already spent on alcohol, cigarettes, and other drugs. One Wednesday night, the couple across the hallway from us threw a roaring party that lasted until two-o'clock in the morning and was followed by a family slugfest. The woman eventually got the man out of their apartment, but he would return every 15 minutes or so, banging on the door and screaming, "I'll kill you,

you bitch!" Repeated visits by the park rangers never seemed to catch the guy when he happened to be assaulting the door.

Next day, we visited the housing office to demand a transfer out of that building.

"Your dorm," the housing administrator assured us, "is by far the most well-behaved residence in the village."

To prove his point, he informed us that at another dorm an employee had just been charged with attempted murder. Somehow, this information didn't ease our concerns.

In addition to the dorm problems, we felt our employer was deliberately taking advantage of desperate people in order to conscript cheap labor and stuff the company coffers. The most telling issue, though, was that Martha and I had precious little time off to pursue the activities that attracted us to the Grand Canyon in the first place: hiking, running, camping, birding, exploring northern Arizona, and re-examining our souls.

In December of 1999, after working the fall season at the Grand Canyon, we paid a ceremonial final visit to the South Rim and stared for the last time into the fathomless depths. Since then, I've always felt as though the Grand Canyon were a part of my own psyche, a wonder of the world I can take with me wherever I go.

After this affectionate farewell, we resumed our wanders throughout the West, in search of something more substantial than the broken American Dream, and something less tangible than the pot at the end of the rainbow.

What we found, after exploring many towns over the next few weeks, was Ashland, Oregon, site of the famous Oregon Shakespeare Festival. It was here, in a region filled with colorful legends and historical ghosts, that we thought we'd discovered our Zen habitation.

Little did we know that a trickster as mischievous as Puck the sprite was waiting to teach us a lesson in self-deception. As the Bard himself once put this proposition, "There are more things in heaven and earth, Horatio, than are dreamt of in your philosophy."

At the Mercy of the Vortex

Ashland is a charming little hamlet filled with quaint Victorian cottages, theatrical characters, and Shakespearean fanatics. Quite literally, "the play's the thing." The residents and visitors take their plays more seriously than anyone this side of 17th-century Stratford-on-Avon.

One time, when a renowned Shakespearean scholar arrived in town for a lecture, he asked to be housed a far cry from the theater district.

"I don't want to be woken at six in the morning," he complained, "by combatants shouting misinformation about Shakespeare."

In fact, I once witnessed just such a shouting match over one of the non-Shakespearean plays being produced at the festival. It happened right after a performance of Edmond Rostand's *Cyrano de Bergerac*, in which the hero's schnoz had been deliberately shortened from its traditional Pinocchio size to a more human Karl Malden dimension.

"My God!" barked the purist, "all the humor and most of the philosophy revolve around Cyrano's outsized nose."

"Bah!" shouted the avant-gardist. "Cyrano's nose is the most overrated stage prop in all theater. He's needed a nose job for a long, long time."

With all its theatrics, Ashland seemed like just the sort of odd and wonderful place where Martha and I could feel at home. After finding an economical motel efficiency with a monthly rate, we spent our time exploring the surrounding countryside, developing a business plan for an Internet antiques dealership to support us, and taking long sojourns through Lithia Park, a former Chautauqua grounds that is probably the prettiest town preserve in the entire country.

When it comes to soul-searching, of course, appearances are often deceiving, mainly because the mind is constantly playing Puckish pranks on itself. It's as if each of us comes equipped with an elfin alter-ego, hiding behind trees and bushes, whose job is to whisper misinformation in our ears.

Martha and I kept saying the same thing, time and time again, about pretty little Ashland: "We ought to love it here." This was Puck, hard at work, whispering in our ears. Meanwhile, we kept denying that in our heart of hearts we were sensing something else entirely.

After a month of deliberating, still operating under the influence of our own mischievous sprites, Martha and I signed a lease, put down a first- and last-month's deposit on a funky little rental cottage, and began preparations to make Ashland our permanent home.

But it didn't work out that way.

First of all, we soon learned it would cost us more than $8,000 to ship all our belongings cross-country from Massachusetts. This fee did much more than put a price tag on our wavering commitment to Ashland. It also gave us pause to consider the high cost of spiritual questing, and the very sanity of this long, strange trip we were on.

Meanwhile, something even more dear than movers' fees was going on below the surface. From the moment we occupied our empty rental house, and for a period of the next three weeks, I didn't sleep. I don't mean I suffered occasional bouts of insomnia, I mean I didn't sleep at all. In a matter of days, I turned into a stoop-shouldered zombie, as sleep deprivation quickly took a toll on both my mood and my blood sugar.

Martha and I made a joke of this episode, blaming my sleeplessness on one of the powerful vortexes for which Oregon is famous, those mysterious anomalies that create both physical and psychic freakishness wherever they exist. It soon became apparent, however, that the vortex located in this house was something not of this earth, but of my spirit.

What it was saying was, "I don't want to live here."

Under Siege by Mallards

As usual, being the soul mates we are, Martha and I reached exactly the same conclusion about Ashland at precisely the same time.

Picture this scene. The only furnishings in our little rental cottage were two folding camp chairs, a wooden crate, two air mattresses, and a portable TV set. Furthermore, whoever had lived here previously must have fed the ducks in the adjacent pond on a regular basis, because the resident mallards kept us in a state of constant siege by quacking outside our windows day and night.

One morning, as the mallards clamored outside and we were sitting in our folding chairs eating breakfast, Martha and I regarded each other thoughtfully. The empty house seemed oppressive. The money we had dumped into signing a lease hung over our heads. The prospect of spending $8,000 on shipping our furniture cross-country and making the final commitment to Ashland weighed on both our minds. The situation was made even more complicated by a sickness in the family back East.

"Where do you feel most at home in the world," I suddenly said above the din of the ducks.

Martha thought for a few seconds.

"Cape Cod," she said.

"Then what are we doing here?" I said.

The answer was obvious. As soon as the thought was spoken, as soon as the words made official what was in our souls, everything instantly fell into place. To paraphrase T. S. Eliot: When you arrive at the beginning once again and know it for the first time, only then will you understand the truth. Having gone full circle in a journey around the entire United States, we were about to arrive at the beginning once more and know it for the first time.

You Can't Get There
from Here

I don't know how this mechanism works, but once you've made a right decision about anything of lasting importance, the universe seems to stretch at your feet like a purring cat. After we made the decision to live on Cape Cod, all the forces of nature lined up behind Martha and myself and, like a powerful trade wind, pushed us across the continent. As we drove through the northern states during the last week of February 2000, an unprecedented high-pressure system accompanied us all the way, keeping the temperatures in the seventies and eighties and setting records from Montana to Chicago.

You are probably asking yourself the same question we kept posing as we floated along in our high-pressure zone. Why hadn't we just gone to Cape Cod in the first place? After all, it's just a three-hour drive from Amherst to the Cape. The answer, as they say in New England, is "You can't get there from here."

I'm still convinced we took the only course, circuitous as it was, that could lead us to Cape Cod. As all tough choices must, this one had to be made the hard way; a picaresque route mapped out by heavenly forces more savvy than human consciousness and running through 11,000 miles of detours, switchbacks, and dead ends.

I have no doubt that, without driving to hell and back, we couldn't have discovered what was in our hearts in the first place. But as exhausting as our trip had been, once we settled on Cape Cod, we knew at once we were where we ought to be.

I won't say our life here has been idyllic, though there are certainly elements of *that*; but I can honestly claim that every day is cathartic. There is something about the irregular coast line of the Cape, with its thousands of picturesque nooks and crannies, that reflects the many shades of my own psyche, giving all my sides a voice they never had before.

Like any other guy with a complex inner life, one that some alienists might term as "neurotic," I am a person of a thousand disguises. Life on Cape Cod proves they're all me.

Live with Passion and Die with Thanks

In many respects, life is a perpetual process of finding oneself. What I'm finding on Cape Cod is worthwhile writing, values that are socially redeeming, a lifestyle that is simplified, relationships that are fruitful, a world view that makes sense, and diabetic maintenance that is effective, healthful, and constant.

Each moment on Cape Cod reminds me how I've totally transformed my life since first being diagnosed with diabetes.

My own method of spiritual trekking has involved a lot of soul-searching, a good deal of reading, the practice of several spiritual techniques (which will be detailed in Part 3), a change of employment, and a pilgrimage to find a new residence that feels like a soulful place to be.

My five-year trek toward self-discovery has taught me optimism, hope, perspective, perseverance, tolerance, passion, joy, zest for life, satisfaction, harmony, well-being, purpose, and a desire to help other people.

I would never be so presumptuous as to suggest that you or anyone else should tread my own crooked road toward self-fulfillment, or follow my own oddball example of self-realization. Each of us must find his or her own kind of transformation. We're all different.

You must become your own Path in your own way.

Or, as one of my former English professors used to say: "Don't hear the bell, be the bell."

Suffice it to say, on Cape Cod I believe I've found the optimum conjunction of gravitational forces, psychic drives, astrological influences, scenic wonders, chemical attractions, spiritual revelations, healthy habits, good vibrations, and whatever other mysterious forces control my stormy behavior.

As for you, you might not even need to move out of your armchair to transform your life. Only you can say for sure.

Let me end my personal story of transformation with a prayer of sorts, summing up the "right conduct" I hope to carry out, now that I've gone through my diabetic baptism by fire. If I don't always live up to the vows I make in the following credo, at least they give me enough worthwhile activities to keep me out of the opium dens, away from the speakeasies, and off the mean streets of Cape Cod.

Promises to Keep

I will value the metaphysical, the otherworldly, the mysterious, and the baffling above all else. I will forgive my own trespasses as I would forgive those who trespass against me. I will look to the demented, the outcast, the forsaken, and the crazed for wisdom. I will despise cell phones, stock markets, reality TV, and war. I will treat ants and spiders and mice as prophets. I will help protect heaven and earth from polluters. I will praise my enemies for teaching me the lessons I most need. I will respect any opinion as long as it is honest, tolerant, and unrehearsed. I will honor eccentrics of every ilk. I will suffer fools gladly. I will disregard official spokespersons everywhere. I will thumb my nose at phonies and bullies. When all else fails, I will give away everything I own. I will accept the past for what it is and change the future to what it should be. I will treat my diabetes with all due respect. I will live with passion and die with thanks.

two

Insulin for the Soul

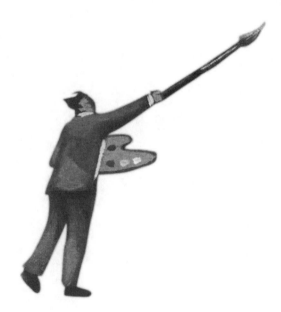

*The Medical
Link Between
Spirituality
and Health*

From the Ass to the Soul
How the Body Relates to the Spirit

Reverend Edward Schroeder, a retired theology professor from St. Louis who also has diabetes, tells a true anecdote about a man admitted to an intensive care unit with a life-threatening illness. During his time flirting with death, the man quickly learned how important his own spirituality was to his recovery.

"You know," the man concluded after he was out of danger, "I came in here to save my ass, and I found out it was connected to my soul."

The pathway between the *gluteus maximus* and the *spiritus humanus*, in essence, is what this book is all about. Likewise, the spirit-body connection is the nitty-gritty of what I've learned the hard way about my diabetes. Trying to save my own ass, I discovered that the arteries of my blood led directly to my soul.

In the fond hope that all of us can save our own asses, Part 2 of *Zen and the Art of Diabetes Maintenance* will answer four key questions about the impact of spiritual belief on health:

- Does medical research indicate that faith, religion, and spiritual practices exert a positive effect on health in general?
- Has the medical community concluded that faith and spirituality have a role to play in the health care of patients, especially those with chronic illnesses?
- Can medical professionals who deal specifically with diabetes observe the positive influence of spirituality on the health and well-being of their patients with diabetes?
- Do those people with diabetes who have deep spiritual beliefs manage their health and their lives better than those without any kind of spirituality?

As you will soon see, the answer to all these questions is affirmative. The researchers, psychologists, medical professionals, and diabetes educators interviewed in this section have determined that the medical community has recently begun to take very seriously the role of spirituality in healing, the power of the mind-body link, and the critical part faith can play in medical care.

I will also show the connection between spirituality and health from the viewpoint of people with diabetes. Later in this section, I will relate the actual stories of people whose diabetes transformed their existence in various ways. In the process, I will tell the stories of people with diabetes who have: led inspirational lives of many kinds; approached their disease management in unorthodox and dramatic ways; revolutionized their metaphysical outlooks; worked for agencies and foundations and projects to improve the human condition; espoused life-enhancing causes; remained optimistic and satisfied in face of terribly debilitating complications; performed amazing athletic feats; and changed their quality of life in all-encompassing fashion, thus making themselves into more productive, more spiritually evolved human beings.

Each in his or her own way, these unassuming role models have discovered the truth of what the Roman wise man Hiraclitus concluded some 500 years before Christ:

"Character is destiny."

All these voices from that sweet beyond called diabetes also echo the prophetic words spoken in the film version of Bernard Malamud's thoughtful baseball novel, *The Natural*:

"I believe we lead two lives. The life we learn with, and the life we live with after that."

One more purpose of Part 2 is to explore the many diverse faces of spirituality, especially as they concern diabetes. Many of us are a lot more spiritual than we think. There are multiple sides to the spirit, and the spirit shows itself in multiple ways. According to Buddha, the ability to realize the naked truth is the ultimate spiritual experience. A feeling of union with nature is a different side of spiritualism, as Thoreau's *Walden* so eloquently expressed. To the scientist, critical observation is a spiritual practice. For the artist, nothing is more spiritual than writing a poem, or creating a sculpture, or composing soaring music. A teacher's definition of spirituality might be the magic moment when the light of curiosity first shines in the eyes of a troubled student. The ability to overcome incredible obstacles is yet one more gift of the human spirit. All these expressions of spirituality, and many more besides, are every bit as valid as the rites of any religion.

One of the most spiritual moments I ever experienced was at the age of 33, when I woke up in my hospital bed and was told I hadn't died from acute pancreatitis. I spent the next seven days focusing all my spirit on healing myself, and it worked. I was later informed that only five percent of patients survive the kind of attack I'd suffered.

Transformation of the Tawdry into the Precious

The fact that spiritual faith has been born again into the practice of medicine is all very surprising, considering that until a few years ago most doctors regarded all connection between spirituality and health as mere superstition. Many medical professionals looked at the healing power of faith in much the same light as they did alchemy.

Alchemy, as you might well know, was a kind of magical chemistry practiced during the Middle Ages, with many spiritual and philosophical associations. Alchemy's stated goal was to change cheap base metals into gold. It that sense, it was one of the early incarnations for the entrepreneurial spirit.

But this transmutation of the tawdry into the precious had much deeper implications, for the transcendent purpose of alchemy was eternal life and perpetual youth. Somewhere buried in the ancient myths and preternatural lore of human culture was the belief that a certain very pure form of gold, when ingested, could confer mastery over death.

When I tripped over the transforming power of my own diabetes, I also lucked into a new kind of alchemy. An alchemy of the soul. The magical chemistry of my blood sugar, which dragged me kicking and screaming into a new way of life, changed my baser instincts into a precious quantity that has given me a glimpse of immortality. Blood-sugar alchemy has released the infinity of my soul. It's a gift more cherished than gold.

Alchemy is a good symbol for the way that modern medicine has traditionally regarded the relationship between spirituality and health. Medicine lumped all beliefs about the power of spiritual healing into the same witch's brew as alchemy, voodoo, and black magic. Now the medical community is slowly beginning to accept the fact that people's deepest spiritual beliefs exercise a profound influence over their health. Science is coming to the same realization that I did, in my own serendipitous style; that an intense spiritual faith can transform one's health and well-being in many deep-seated ways.

"I believe that the evidence is clear," Herbert Benson M.D. said in his book *Timeless Healing: The Power and Biology of Belief*. "Our bodily systems enjoy the results of our wiring, faith coursing through us with tremendous influence. With a visceral, inseparable soul and a genetic predisposition to sooth ourselves, we can better cope with the daily strain of life and more fully appreciate the great Mystery of it all. Faith affirms life, perpetually and timelessly."

Searching for the Ultimate Welfare State

As you will read on the following pages, the scientific evidence for the health-giving qualities of spirituality are becoming overwhelming, both quantitatively and anecdotally. At the same time, the medical definition of healthfulness is expanding to meet the demands of a health-conscious society.

"Health is our natural state," said spiritual writer Deepak Chopra M.D. in his book *Creating Health: Beyond Prevention, Toward Perfection*. "The World Health Organization has defined it as something more than the absence of disease or infirmity. Health is the state of perfect physical, mental, and social well-being. To this may be added spiritual well-being, a state in which a person feels at every moment of living a joy and zest for life, a sense of fulfillment, and an awareness of harmony with the universe."

How do sensitive souls respond to a brave new world in which selfishness is consecrated, compassion is ridiculed, money is deified, and our cultural icons act deeply shallow?

As football Hall-of-Famer Knute Rockne said about the shallow society: "Most people, when they think they are thinking, are merely rearranging their prejudices."

In a society where life imitates TV, thoughtful people will eventually search for something more substantial. They will look for a kind of "welfare state," in the transcendent sense of that term, where overall healthfulness is something quite deliberate and holistic, rather than an accident of nature.

"It is the mind," said 19th-century abolitionist Sojourner Truth, "that makes the body."

Is Religion Good for
Your Health?

The Research of Dr. Harold G. Koenig

One of the foremost experts on the research surrounding spirituality and health is Dr. Harold Koenig, M.D., who is founder and director of the Center for the Study of Religion/ Spirituality and Health at Duke University Medical Center. He has written more than 150 scientific articles, 35 book chapters, and 14 books on subjects related to spirituality and health, including his groundbreaking work, *The Handbook of Religion and Health*, an 800-page reference manual that deals with 1,200 research studies on the topic.

The essence of Dr. Koenig's work can be found in the title of his 1997 book: *Is Religion Good for Your Health?* His answer to this overarching question is unequivocal.

"About two-thirds of the studies, or 800 of 1,200, show a statistically significant connection between religion and good health," Dr. Koenig says. "It doesn't necessarily mean that religion is causing good health. What it means is that religiously involved people appear to be healthier, both physically and mentally, and don't need as many health services, as non-involved individuals."

Why does his center focus more on research measuring organized religious practices than the spirituality that ought to be any religion's inspiration? His answer voices a practical concern for doing any scientific study on the connection between faith and health: Spirituality is essentially unquantifiable.

That's why much of the research about the effects of spirituality on health uses traditional religious practices, such as attendance at services or scripture reading, as the units of measurement for quantifying the studies. Thus, many of these studies deal more with people active in religious groups than with people, such as myself, who exercise our spirit unilaterally. Why? Because we practice something less measurable, though no less important, than religion.

The Helper's High and Other Healthful Mechanisms

Despite restricting his survey to the quantifiable aspects of faith, Dr. Koenig's summary of the research makes a graceful argument for the health benefits of spirituality and religion. Here are some of his conclusions about religious (and presumably spiritual) people and their health, as compared to non-believers and their health. Religious people:

- have significantly lower diastolic blood pressure
- are hospitalized less often
- are less likely to suffer depression
- have healthier lifestyles
- have a stronger sense of well-being and life satisfaction
- have significantly better health outcomes after being stricken with illnesses
- have stronger immune systems
- live longer
- are better protected from cardiovascular disease and cancer

What is the physical mechanism for this spirit-body link? According to Dr. Koenig, faith and religious practices exert many influences on the emotional and biological pathways through which the mind affects the body. They improve mental health, which in turn positively influences the immune system, the autonomic nervous system, and the release of stress hormones. Religious activity increases social support, which in turn encourages more preventive behavior related to disease detection and treatment compliance. And spiritual people tend to avoid habits that could be detrimental to their health, such as smoking, alcohol abuse, risky sexual behavior, and drug use.

Anyone with a modicum of medical knowledge about diabetes can see how the entire mechanism, as described above, also translates to better blood-sugar management.

With all this in mind, what is the best possible attitude for dealing with a chronic illness such as diabetes?

"I can answer that with as much certainty as I am able to answer any question," Dr. Koenig says. "The most important factor is when people with chronic illness reach out to others and offer spiritual encouragement, moral support, social service, and volunteer assistance. That right there is, in a nutshell, the key to people being successful in coping with chronic illness."

Dr. Koenig's comments about helping behavior recall the research of Dr. Allan Luks, former director of the Institute for the Advancement of Health, who surveyed 1,000 volunteers across the nation. Dr. Luks discovered that volunteers engaged in helping other people consistently report better health than peers in their own age group. He called this phenomenon "The Helper's High." Eighty to 95 percent of those surveyed reported that helping behavior gave them a physical rush, more energy, a sense of euphoria, long-term relaxation, and/or a permanent ripple effect of wellness whenever they recalled their volunteer efforts in later years.

"It is one of the beautiful compensations of this life," said Charles Dudley Warner, "that no one can sincerely try to help another without helping oneself."

Dr. Koenig's scientific work on how religion and spirituality impact health seems to form a firm, objective foundation for my own very subjective discoveries about the healing power of the soul. As the research indicates, spirituality and faith tend to bless religious practitioners with a sense of purpose that overcomes many physical disabilities, either directly through better health, or indirectly through healing of the spirit.

"My case is clear," Dr. Koenig says about his survey of the research. "There is no doubt that, rather than feeling depressed and hopeless over a chronic disease like diabetes, if you have a sense of spiritual purpose and meaning, of course you're going to take better care of yourself. I've seen that over and over again."

The Forgotten Factor in Medicine

Dr. David B. Larson and His Findings About Spirituality

D r. David Larson, president of the International Center for the Integration of Health and Spirituality, is one of the leading researchers and lecturers in the country on the subject of spirituality and health. He speaks at 30 to 40 medical conferences each year that deal with what he calls the "spiritual dimension," which, until a few years ago, he considered "the forgotten factor in medicine."

"It's not forgotten anymore, as the scores of conferences dealing with it would indicate," Dr. Larson says. "The movement in medicine to consider spirituality and health has become a surprising and, for me, staggering phenomenon. Now we need to get into the specific realm of chronic illnesses such as diabetes. These are the areas where a patient's spirituality can be very relevant to health and coping with illness."

Dr. Larson told me about several key mechanisms by which spirituality might influence the health of people in general, and people with diabetes in particular. For example, the social support present in spiritual groups is one valuable mechanism, since this type of positive reinforcement can help people with diabetes and other patients manage their illnesses better. Spirituality can also improve patients' coping skills by giving them the positive, can-do attitude that is so closely linked to deep spiritual belief. In addition, it can affect personal lifestyle, with spiritually inclined people tending to treat themselves in more healthful ways than non-spiritual people. And metaphysical beliefs can help the mind-body relationship through the positive psychology inspired by such spiritual practices as love, forgiveness, and gratitude.

"These can all be life-enhancing behaviors," says Dr. Larson about the mechanisms above. "These all create a sense of hope and optimism, which in turn can help people deal better with diabetes and other chronic illness."

Dr. Schroeder, the theologist mentioned previously, has reached the same conclusion as Dr. Larson, but from his own perspective as a spiritually involved person with diabetes.

"I guess my own attitude about health goes back to having an optimistic approach to life, coming to the conclusion I am healed in my own way," he says. "I might be incurable, but I'm not desperate. It's clearly true, and well-documented in medical studies, that a positive approach and sense of well-being are much more healthful when dealing with chronic illnesses than a negative approach and sense of hopelessness."

Emily Dickinson expressed this same concept, through a religious experience called poetry, more than a century ago:

Hope is the thing with feathers
That perches in the soul,
And sings the tune without the words,
And never stops at all.

The Guilt That Keeps on Gifting

Don't let me leave you with the false impression that all religion produces hope and optimism in its practitioners and that all religious practice is good for your health. Dr. Larson quotes Garrison Keillor on the guilt practiced so religiously by so many spiritual groups over the ages: "Guilt is the gift that keeps on giving."

And guilt is just one of the bad attitudes that impact health when religious extremists break faith with their own medical treatment.

"Some people have negative religion," says Dr. Larson. "The norm is that religion creates a more positive viewpoint toward life. But we're always concerned with the 3–5% of patients who develop negative reactions, such as guilt, due to their religious convictions."

Some religious patients look at illness as a kind of almighty punishment. They might actually lose their faith over their fear of divine retribution, which, in turn, can create a negative impact on their health.

"They approach their illness with negative spiritual coping," Dr. Larson explains. "They seem to be saying, 'Here we go. God screwed me again.'"

Those of us who talk to many people with diabetes can always spot the ones who suffer from the "God screwed me again" syndrome. You can almost see a symbolic Scarlet D worn on their chests.

Research recently conducted by Dr. Koenig and Dr. Kenneth Pargament of Bowling Green State University clearly demonstrates Dr. Larson's concern about "negative religion." Their study was based on a questionnaire and a two-year follow-up study of 600 patients, all over the age of 55, at Duke University Medical Center. The study's questionnaire ended up raising three notable red flags about patients' religious attitudes:

- those who "wondered whether God had abandoned me" later exhibited a 28% increased risk of dying
- those who "questioned God's love for me" showed a 22% increased risk
- those who "decided the devil made this happen" suffered from a 19% increased risk

"By looking at both negative and positive factors," says Dr. Larson, "this needed study more specifically investigated various aspects of spirituality that may have harmful health consequences for increasing mortality risk. More studies are needed to better understand the 'dark side' of spiritual and religious commitment."

Another unhealthy religious behavior is substituting religion for health care, a custom practiced by sects that counsel their believers to avoid medical treatment. The perfect example was reported on *60 Minutes* with the case of Lorie and Dennis Nixon, members of a fundamentalist denomination in Altoona, Pennsylvania, that regards medical intervention as an offense against the sect's rigid religious code.

In 1996, the Nixons' 16-year-old daughter went into a diabetic coma and never responded to the family's ritualistic prayer, which they substituted for traditional medicine. After their daughter died, the Nixons were charged with, and convicted of, involuntary manslaughter, their second such conviction. Another child, an eight-year-old boy, had died in 1992 of a common ear infection after his parents refused medical treatment for their child.

Dr. Larson also warns against those well-documented religious cults that destroy their members' health and well-being in numerous ways, using such techniques as brain-washing, social isolation, peer pressure, and group paranoia. There are numerous negative outcomes from these belief-driven approaches to medical care, even death.

Possibly the most tragic case of unhealthy cult activity was the infamous incident at Jonestown, Guyana, in which nearly the entire congregation of the Reverend James Jones died from Kool-Aid laced with cyanide.

"Jones and his cult served as the perfect example of harmful religious beliefs," says Dr. Larson. "That kind of religion is no good for anybody's health, especially if the followers end up dead."

In essence, health care professionals need to help guide their patients along the hopeful channels of their religious belief systems, while steering them away from the "dark side" of faith. As the old pop song goes, they've got to "accentuate the positive."

"We don't want to be giving spiritually troubled patients negative reinforcement," says Dr. Larson. "We want to take advantage of the resources in spirituality that make believers optimistic about the future."

Burn, Baby, Burn

Perspectives from Craig M. Broadhurst,
Diabetes Educator

As it turned out, negative religion was the key factor in an alarming incident that happened to writer, counselor, and diabetes educator Craig Broadhurst in a North Carolina diabetes clinic several years ago. As soon as Broadhurst entered the treatment room, her new patient looked up and screamed, "I hope this hospital burns down with my doctor in it!"

Broadhurst, who currently practices in Greensboro, North Carolina, where she works as a clinical specialist for the on-line Web site *childrenwithdiabetes.com*, responded in just the right way for a professional counselor. She let the woman cool down before talking with her about the reasons for her flammable feelings.

As Broadhurst later learned, the patient was apparently furious about a free trip to Hawaii she had just lost due to her diabetic complications. But the underlying problem, as the woman was soon able to articulate, was a deep-rooted spiritual crisis. She had lost the religious faith she felt she needed to deal with her diabetes.

Broadhurst's patient had evidently reached a point in her life when she couldn't deal any more with her own diabetes. She had lost that feathery thing called hope, perching in her soul, and was in dire need of perspective, distance, and meaning.

"I think diabetes and chronic disease in general can narrow your vision substantially, to where you forget your place in the world," Broadhurst says. "It can make you forget that it's not just about diabetes. It's about the fact that you have a journey to take, and diabetes is only a part of that journey."

One of Broadhurst's biggest jobs as a diabetes counselor is to help people come to grips with the emotional crisis posed by chronic illness.

"My approach," Broadhurst says, "is to let people tell me as best they can what they're struggling with in terms of their relationship with the universe. I basically try to find out if they think they've fallen off God's radar screen."

One person with diabetes who felt she was well beyond radar range was a woman who had suddenly gained 80 pounds, for no apparent reason. Of course, any astute therapist, such as Broadhurst, understands there's no such thing as "no apparent reason."

The woman's doctor came to Broadhurst and said, "I don't know what's wrong with her. The wheels have come off her management. Fix her."

He might have issued much the same instructions to his mechanic after his BMW developed an alarming noise in the rear axle. But Broadhurst understood from her long experience as a counselor that this was not just a body vexed by a mechanical gremlin. This was a person with a critical psychological issue.

What Broadhurst eventually learned through counseling sessions was that the woman had recently been raped. Her alarming weight gain was a defense mechanism so she wouldn't have to go through that kind of ordeal again. Counseling ultimately gave the patient the spiritual perspective and faith to deal with the horror of her rape and manage her diabetes better.

Broadhurst firmly believes that spirituality is one of the most powerful tools for patients healing themselves, and in many different ways.

"I have come to the conclusion as a therapist dealing with all areas of chronic disease management over the past 18 years," she says, "that for people of faith a spiritual approach to illness is just as important as anything they can do. They tend to optimize both their immune systems and their ability to fight off complications. They tend to manage their illnesses longer, better, and more thoroughly than people who see themselves as victims of disease. That's what I believe."

The Walking-Around-Numb Crowd

When you get right down to it, spirituality is all about feeling: feeling the blessed sensations of nature operating around you; feeling your own inner impulses and compulsions; feeling your own soul breathing inside your body; feeling the creative spirit of your own being; feeling the secret inspiration of life itself.

In that context, Broadhurst gets very passionate about so many people who are "walking around numb," as she puts it.

"By that I mean being an amoeba and not really feeling the gift of life," she says. "That is, until something bad happens. Until they have a life-changing experience such as diabetes. Diabetes wakes up a lot of people."

Having experienced diabetes slapping me in the face, I understand what the healthy reaction should be to this cosmic wake-up call. Shake out the cobwebs and say, "Thanks! I needed that."

"Doctors and patients are supposed to be partners in diabetes management," says Broadhurst. "But I believe faith is also an essential partner. If you go through all the daily grind of management, and stick your fingers, and take your insulin, and go for your walk, but your soul is in despair, it isn't going to work. You also need a belief system that inspires you to control your diabetes."

Can't Win for Losing

"Those who do not hope to win have already lost," said 19th-century Ecuadoran poet José Joaquín de Olmedo.

In this case, the scientific seems to back up the poetic. Hope is one of the key ingredients in developing a belief system that inspires people with diabetes to control their condition. A study in the July/August 2001 issue of *Endocrine Practice,* the medical journal of the American Association of Clinical Endocrinologists, demonstrates that such optimistic attitudes as hope, positive motivation, and a sense of control exert a direct influence over the physical health of people with diabetes.

"The data showed that the more positive the attitude toward the illness," says Kay McFarland, MD, the author of the study, "the better the patient's mental and physical health."

Her study, entitled *Meaning of Illness and Health Outcomes in Type I Diabetes*, showed a direct relationship between the meaning, whether positive or negative, that people with diabetes attribute to their illness and the long-term seriousness of that illness. Dr. McFarland's findings indicate a need for both behavioral and psychological adjustments by people with diabetes. Beyond the behavioral changes related to nutritional modifications and blood-sugar monitoring that people with diabetes routinely make, they need to develop more optimistic, well-motivated attitudes to deal with the stress of living with their chronic illness.

As many medical professionals have discovered, people with diabetes need to exercise a high degree of both physical and emotional control over their condition.

"This study clearly establishes a direct connection between mental and physical health," says Dr. McFarland, "in that *meaning of illness* [my italics] by the patient influences the patient's health outcomes, such as complications."

Bing Bang Bing, Goodbye

*Paula S. Yutzy's 19 Years
Working with Diabetes*

The reality of most diabetic health care is a six- to ten-minute appointment with a primary care physician once every quarter. How often have you finished your regular diabetic checkup, which is over seconds after the doctor glances perfunctorily at your carefully compiled blood-sugar journal, and asked yourself, "Is that all there is?"

Welcome to the Diabetic Division of The "Is That All There Is?" Society, whose theme song of the same name was a popular hit by singer Peggy Lee, nearly a half-century ago.

"Wonderful as that doctor might be," says Paula Yutzy, director of Diabetes Education for the Diabetes Center at Mercy Medical Center in Baltimore, "the bottom line is it's bing bang bing, goodbye, see you in three months. That kind of approach often doesn't work when diabetes is a condition you have to live with 24 hours a day, seven days a week, and it's something you have to face within your own being."

That's where diabetes educators and counselors come in. Quite often, their interventions have nothing to do with the physical manifestations of diabetes. Their job, in many cases, is probing the subtle symptoms of lost faith itself.

"We tend to get far too medical and forget the human side of chronic disease," Yutzy says. "It's not a body that has diabetes, it's a person. It involves the whole personhood, from family relationships to belief systems and everything. It really gets down to inspiration. What can people with diabetes find in their world view that gives them the inspiration to deal with diabetes?"

The Slam-Bam-Thank-You-Ma'am Doctor's Appointment

Getting at this form of inspiration takes a lot more effort than your average slam-bam-thank-you-Ma'am doctor's appointment. That's why many progressive diabetes centers, such as the one at Mercy Medical, give people with diabetes options for consultations that deal more in soul-searching than in finger pricking or exchange lists.

Yutzy and many other diabetes counselors have learned that effective intervention first must soothe the savage soul of a person with diabetes before carrying out the lifelong work of de-sugaring the savage bloodstream.

Counselors must help people with diabetes reach "mature and life-giving conclusions," as Yutzy says. "Of those persons with diabetes who have come to a deeper spiritual awareness, they definitely find that spiritual beliefs inspire them to manage their blood sugar better and, beyond that, to cultivate healthier lifestyles. They find their power from a more total understanding and deal with their lives in a much more healthy manner."

The Wages of a Disorganized Life

"A disorganized life," Yutzy says, "creates disastrous diabetic management."

And what, you might want to ask, serves to organize any life? Only a well-conceived world view. Only a well-disposed viewpoint on creation.

"Spirituality helps people with diabetes," says Yutzy, "because spiritual people are comfortable with their place in the world, and they see diabetes as just part of their lives. They deal with diabetes because they are dealing with everything else in kind. They do it gracefully and unobtrusively. They take it all in stride."

How to Live Graciously with Uncertainty

Observations on Healing from Dr. Valerie Yancey

"Medicine's biggest problem is uncertainty," says Valerie Yancey, director of the Holistic Nursing Masters Program at the Jewish Hospital School of Nursing and Allied Health at Washington University School of Medicine in St. Louis. "If we knew for sure how things were going to end, there wouldn't be any need for soul-searching. But we don't. So, facing chronic illness such as diabetes takes a tremendous store of courage and community support and comfort."

In that respect, as Yancey says, the whole point of facing any serious illness is "to learn how to live graciously with uncertainty."

These surprisingly simple words suggest incredibly complex implications. How does one learn such grace under fire? According to Yancey, it involves a paradoxical course of stick-to-it-ism and letting go.

"In many ways we have to buck up and hang on," Yancey says. "Hang on, hang on, hang on. And there is something blessed about that optimistic, in-your-face coping. But at the same time, we have to recognize that we are powerless in wake of some circumstances, and we have to accept that, too. If we've done the best we can, we can't do any more. That paradox to me is what the healing adventure is all about."

Everybody Dies

I can second her opinion. As a person with diabetes, I've learned that I must live boldly with my disease, doing everything humanly possible to manage it in a gutsy manner. But, at the same time, I have to accept that someday I'll die, as everyone on earth does. I have to fight like hell for life and simultaneously let it go. I do so by envisioning the greater good beyond my own humble existence.

There was an amazingly poignant interview with paralyzed actor Christopher Reeves that beautifully expressed the dovetailing attitudes of hanging on and letting go. Reeves was asked if he thought he would ever walk again.

"I believe there's a very good chance I will walk again," he said, referring to the many advances in spinal chord medicine.

"But what if you can't?" came the follow-up question.

"Then I won't walk again," he said with a tone of perfect acceptance, perfect peace of mind. I have to believe his attitude comes from the wellspring of acceptance, hope, and optimism that bubbles up from spirituality and the way it works in our lives.

Trusting in Synchronicity

Yancey believes she sees God's grace at work whenever the right people seem to be put in the right place at the right time to create a kind of spiritual synchronicity. Perhaps this synchronicity is what Kierkegaard was referring to when he spoke of our ability to understand life only when looking at it backwards. Trusting in synchronicity is what the life of the spirit is all about, Yancey explains, and what healing means. And it exerts many forces on the fate of human health.

"I see spirituality impacting health in several ways," Yancey says. "I see it in spiritual people's wisdom about what is good for their bodies and what isn't. I see it in their serenity. Not complacency, mind you, but more of a willingness to accept what's unfolding. I also see it in the tremendous fight that some people have.

"And then there is the whole question of hope. I see hope as an incredible gift of the spirit that keeps pulling us into God's future by whatever graces come to us. The starting place is knowing that we're all part of this whole plan."

You can see all these forces of faith, serenity, fight, optimism, wisdom, and hope at play in the following chapters, which tell the true stories of people with diabetes who are using the link between spirituality and health to transform their lives.

Writer Napoleon Hill once expressed the power derived from such belief in a universal intelligence this way:

"[Spirituality] restores health where all else fails, in open defiance of all the rules of modern science. It heals the wounds of sorrow and disappointment regardless of their cause."

Reverend Edward Schroeder
God, Guts, and Existentialism

Controlling diabetes, rather than having it control him, could be the major theme of the Reverend Dr. Edward Schroeder's diabetes maintenance over the last 52 years. You can trace his original attitude, when he was diagnosed with diabetes in 1950, at age 19, to his early flirtation with Kierkegaardian existentialism.

"As an existentialist, I accepted that life is one big pain in the ass from beginning to end," he says from his home in St. Louis. "Besides that, I was a Depression baby. I knew I was bound to get mine in one way or another, so my mindset was to stop griping and deal with it."

Born in 1930 in an Illinois farmhouse that has now been in the Schroeder family for more than a century, young Edward was the first of seven German-Lutheran children who grew up in a home atmosphere of strict religion, hard work, and serious baking, although not necessarily in that order.

"I was always a barn-burner," he says, "so when I graduated in three years from my local high school, which had only 64 kids, it wasn't hard to be valedictorian in my class of 14."

The local Lutheran pastor convinced Schroeder's father that Edward should be the first person in his family to attend college. In this case, that meant the nearest Lutheran school, Valparaiso University in Indiana.

Living the Egghead Life

Schroeder was a senior philosophy major there in the winter of 1950, living the "egghead" life of an existentialist, as he puts it, a lifestyle mindful of writer Albert Camus' idea that "Integrity has no need of rules." After taking a nose dive off a toboggan, he proved that one rule he couldn't disobey was the Law of Gravity. When he finally came down, landing right on his sense of integrity, he suffered a mild brain concussion.

Schroeder still believes that his case of diabetes, which was diagnosed several weeks later, had something to do with that blow to the head.

"The doctors all pooh-poohed that theory, of course," says Schroeder. "I now understand that there are more mysteries about diabetes than answers, even if the doctors do all sound like know-it-alls."

In 1950, the short-lived fate of most people with diabetes was a foregone conclusion, but such dire predictions never fazed Schroeder. He proceeded to live a long life bursting with optimism, especially for a budding young existentialist. After graduating from Valparaiso, he attended Concordia Lutheran Seminary in St. Louis and married a professor's daughter. He followed his wife to Germany, where she went on a Fulbright Scholarship, and earned his doctorate in theology at the University of Hamburg.

Since then he has labored diligently at becoming a widely published author, a theology professor at Valparaiso, Concordia, and Christ Seminary-Seminex, and a Lutheran mission volunteer in Australia, Ethiopia, Brazil, Indonesia, Lithuania, and other places.

"I've worked on all the continents except Antarctica," he says with his usual dry humor, "where the Lutherans really haven't gotten a foothold yet."

Juvenile Onset Existentialism

Though Schroeder did a lot of globe trotting, he didn't bring much old baggage with him, such as any fear of his type 1 diabetes, for example, or any pessimism inspired by the juvenile onset existentialism he flirted with as a college kid.

"My life has been frightfully full," he says. "I've been well-traveled, I've had the chance to teach all over the place. Diabetes hasn't inhibited me from living a wonderful life. I've somehow incorporated it into my routine, although it's often been a chore. But it has never stopped me from doing anything I really wanted to do."

That includes munching on the sumptuous baked goods he learned to love as a farm boy, where the sweet aromas of his mother's pies and cakes routinely filled the house. In fact, Schroeder calls his sweet tooth, which he regularly feeds with his own baking, "the biggest challenge in managing my diabetes."

How has Schroeder managed to defy all the experts, who never expected him to reach the age of 40, even though he still takes a healthy helping of dessert now and again? He attributes it to one word, "optimism," a term not often linked to the existentialism he romanced as a youth.

"My gut feeling is that your body is definitely connected to your soul," he says. "I've reached the age of 70, and I'm in relatively good health. I've not yet been cured of diabetes, and I don't anticipate I will before I die. But I'm already healed. As a whole person, I'm okay."

Part of his spiritual healing and physical well-being can be attributed to the good old standbys of diabetes maintenance: regular exercise, good blood-sugar management, eating right, being of good cheer, staying busy at a job he loves, and relating to the "interesting people" that are his passion.

But he also has a hunch about another healthful factor, one proven by the medical research cited previously—the supportive power of a spiritual community.

"I suspect there are some people praying for my survival," he says. "I believe that one reason I've stayed alive so long is the invisible community of people who care for me. That community would include the folks from all the places where I've taught and pastored all over the world. These are blessings that aren't easily explicable."

Michael Jessup
Walking Miracle

On April 17, 1999, five days after his diabetes-related pancreas transplant, Michael Jessup was in trouble. His new pancreas had sent his kidney into shock, his rejection treatment had triggered fever, vomiting, and brain swelling, and he was on a ventilator in the intensive care unit at The Johns Hopkins Hospital in Baltimore. Jessup, who was 34 at the time, had never been a religious man in the traditional sense, but he was deeply spiritual in his own way.

"I wasn't doing very well," he says, "and I was by myself in ICU. So I just said to the guy upstairs, 'You know, I've done everything I can. Now I need a little help.' When I woke up next morning, everything was fine, and two days later I was out of the hospital.

So I can honestly say somebody's been watching over me."

Jessup, who was diagnosed with diabetes at the age of nine, hasn't needed an insulin shot since that operation. For a lad who wasn't supposed to reach the age of 30, and who had been hovering near death for two years prior to the operation, he can now look forward to a long and productive life.

"A lot of people consider me a walking miracle," Jessup says from his office at Salisbury State University in Maryland, where he is the director of annual giving.

Jessup believes the miracle, in this instance, is as much spiritual as it is medical. As thousands of people with diabetes are finding out: What we believe is what we are.

That's when His Bladder Burst

Jessup's story really began shortly before his ninth birthday, while he was trying on a baseball glove in a sporting goods store. That's when his bladder burst. By the time he arrived at the hospital, his blood sugar was 1,150. He still considers that moment strike one in his life.

"I will never forget overhearing the doctor tell my parents outside my hospital room that my life expectancy was about 30," he says. "It was from that day on that I decided I was going to beat diabetes. I might die from old age, or get hit by a golf ball, or fall to some other act of God, but I was not going to give in to this disease."

Jessup considers himself lucky that his parents treated him just like any other kid. He grew up keeping his blood sugars under control through insulin, diet, and exercise, and led a relatively normal life until he was past 30, long enough to prove that doctor, the one overheard outside his hospital room when he as nine, dead wrong.

Then complications set in.

In 1995, Jessup developed diabetic retinopathy and ultimately went through eight surgeries on his right eye and five on his left. But that was just the beginning. On February 26, 1997, just 24 hours after he and his wife Kim listened to the heartbeat of their unborn daughter for the first time, Jessup learned he was suffering from end-stage renal disease. The prognosis related to his failing kidneys was that he might not live to see his daughter born. That was strike two.

But Jessup fooled the experts again. By staying mentally strong, never giving up, and using his daughter's upcoming birth as his inspiration, he hung on. About two months after his daughter Emily was born in September of 1997, Jessup received the "gift of life," a kidney transplant, from his brother Mark.

"There's still a part of me that still does not comprehend how somebody can do that for somebody else," he says about his brother's sacrifice.

The Judas Kiss

But Jessup was still not out of the woods. His blood sugar continued to plant its Judas kiss on the rest of his organs. The day after his kidney transplant,

Jessup was placed on the list for a pancreas transplant, which eventually happened some 15 months later, on April 12, 1999.

"When I woke up in ICU after the operation," Jessup says, "my dream of awakening one morning without diabetes had finally come true." He had swung at strike three, sailing high and hard over the heart of the plate, and smacked it over the fence.

"At Johns Hopkins, they will tell you to this day," Jessup says. "They do not know how I lasted as long as I have. The only conclusion they've reached is that I mentally fought it off. My attitude, ever since I was diagnosed, was diabetes is never going to kill me."

As one result of his attitude, Jessup has spent much of his spare time since his resurrection from the dead doing public speaking to diabetes groups, visiting dialysis units, lecturing to medical students, working on the board of the American Diabetes Association, and raising money for causes, such as the National Kidney Foundation. He is living proof of the "helper's high" and the salubrious benefits of volunteer work.

Counting his blessings is part of that high. Jessup passes a lot of his time while walking on beaches, playing golf, or sitting in empty churches by reflecting on his miraculous comeback.

"Diabetes has absolutely helped me evolve as a spiritual human being," he says about the catalyst for so much in his life. "I am the person I am today because of my diabetes, because of my transplants, because of the perspective I developed from being sick. That's what created me today."

Rod Frantz

Real Men Are Type 1

Forty-seven-year-old Rod Frantz, the assistant director of Pittsburgh's Riverlife Task Force, would certainly agree with Michael Jessup that diabetes makes a person evolve as a human being. But Frantz goes even further than that.

"Diabetes drives you to go through incredible life changes," Frantz says from his home in Pittsburgh, "changes that you wouldn't make except by brute force. Nobody goes there voluntarily."

Frantz sums up the toughening effect of his juvenile onset diabetes in his typically witty style: "Real men are type 1."

Indeed, Frantz considers his own job as a good metaphor for the revolutionary changes he has endured. He is currently helping Pittsburgh through the same kind of total transformation he was forced to make because of his type 1 diabetes.

The Riverlife Task Force is a nonprofit organization dedicated to the rediscovery and re-utilization of Pittsburgh's rivers and river fronts, thus redirecting the whole future of the city. The task force is all part of the city's revitalization struggle, due in no small part to the demise of its traditional heavy industry and the breakdown of the region's economic and social structure. When its steel economy faltered, Pittsburgh lost more industrial base than any Western city since the firebombing of Dresden.

A Paralyzing State of Dislocation

Frantz sums up these problems as Pittsburgh's "paralyzing state of dislocation." Historically speaking, Pittsburgh's troubles resemble those of Frantz, after diabetes caused a paralyzing state of dislocation in his own personal life.

Brought up in Pittsburgh, Frantz left home at the age of 17, suffering from a major case of alienation brought on by diabetes. In effect, he had been firebombed by his own blood sugar.

His early years as a person with diabetes were shaped largely by the negative attitude passed on by much of the medical establishment in the bad old days, when brow-beating, guilt trips, and scare tactics were the main orientation techniques used on so many people newly diagnosed with diabetes. After being diagnosed at the age of eight, Frantz was told he would never live very long and was subjected to the usual gauntlet of damaging remarks.

One doctor asked him, "Do you know why there is a much lower incidence of diabetes in the Soviet Union than in the United States?" When young Frantz shook his head, the doctor answered: "Because they don't let people with diabetes breed there."

"Well, I remembered all those insensitive and, one might even say, mean-spirited remarks," says Frantz now, "and they shaped my own attitude for the early years of my life. That kind of experience certainly formed the underlying philosophy of nihilism and hopelessness that caused me to become an alcoholic."

Suffering from chronic feelings of resentment and abandonment, Frantz left Pittsburgh after his high school graduation and never looked back. He attended college at American University in Washington, D.C., where he later earned his B.A. in communications, formed a successful rock band called the Urban Vervs, and started a hipster hot spot named the 9:30 Club. In accordance with his new lifestyle, his diabetes management basically amounted to a steady diet of sex, drugs, and rock & roll. And not to forget booze. By his own admission, Frantz was aiming to live out his short but eventful life in a blaze of glory.

But his wild life gradually changed with his marriage to a good woman, the birth of his two sons, and his own spiritual resurrection. All those events led him to Alcoholics Anonymous, where he discovered a powerful version of divine salvation and mystical synchronicity, one that he could finally relate to.

A God of Your Own Understanding

"I've never felt entirely at ease with Christianity or organized religion," he says. "But, at the same time, from a very early point in my life, I've believed there was a power greater than myself. The AA concept of 'a God of your own understanding' really resonated with me, and the whole experience carried over into my management of diabetes. I stopped drinking, I stopped smoking, I stopped doing drugs; all the rebellious activities I'd engaged in as the leader of a rock-and-roll band."

Echoing all the research cited earlier in this section about the impact of a positive approach to chronic illness, Frantz says that, "My spiritual rebirth gave me the optimism to face my diabetes problem and overcome it."

But he had one last quest to carry out before completing his personal crusade. He still needed to cure his long-term feeling of rootlessness and lack of direction.

"Now my revolution led me back to my roots in Pittsburgh," says Frantz, "and the kind of humanitarian work I'm involved with now. I soon found that both Pittsburgh and myself were taking the same positive direction after our dislocation. What we're undertaking with the Riverlife Task Force is spiritually analogous to my own journey of understanding."

Frantz likes to call his own pilgrimage his Shining Path, a term he shamelessly borrowed from Far Eastern politics, though without the political connotations.

"My life has definitely been on a path," he says, "and that path has led me from having what I considered an absolutely hopeless medical condition, to the point now, where I am managing my diabetes quite effectively and pouring my heart and soul into this Riverlife Task Force."

Where will his Shining Path take him in the future? After the Riverlife Task Force runs its course, he plans to become a certified diabetes educator and teach others the hard lessons he's had to learn on his own.

"I've always wanted to do something that left the world a slightly better place than when I found it," he says. "I know I'm doing that by raising children who are respectful and creative and a force for good. Certainly working with the Riverlife Task Force is another. You can't overstate the force for good diabetes has played in my life. Certainly, that's a Shining Path."

Vicki Gaubeca

People with Diabetes Strike Back!

Like many people with diabetes I've talked to, much of Vicki Gaubeca's attitude about life has been formed by her reactions, both positive and negative, to key medical professionals she has met along the way.

When Gaubeca was a teenager, growing up in her native Mexico City, she was doing a lot of swimming and biking to help control her recently diagnosed juvenile diabetes, and she would often experience low blood sugar during her exercising. So she went to her family physician and told him, "I think you need to lower my insulin."

The doctor was a member in good standing of the "Father Knows Best" school of physicians and told young Vicki, in effect, that her knowledge of insulin dosages was full of hogwash. The very next day, she suffered a severe hypoglycemic reaction and subsequently began lowering her insulin dosages herself.

"That was the first time I ever took the initiative to follow my own instincts and experiences," she says from her office at the Arizona Health Sciences Center in Tucson, where she works as an editor in the Public Affairs Office. Gaubeca has been taking her own initiative ever since.

Later, when she was in her mid-twenties, Gaubeca met a nurse with diabetes who changed her life in a positive way. Meeting this nurse was a watershed moment, because she showed Gaubeca her own diary and the fluctuations in her own blood glucose level, which weren't too different from Vicki's sugar readings. The nurse, in essence, convinced Gaubeca to have compassion for herself, to educate herself about diabetes, and to do the best she could under the circumstances.

"Until then," she recalls, "it was typical for me to go to a doctor and have him chew me out because I wasn't controlling my diabetes, which at that time was very difficult to do with the methodology of the seventies and eighties. I now understand that it's nearly impossible for a type 1 to control the condition using an intermediate insulin that has its peaks at unpredictable times."

The Seven Deadly Sins of Doctors

Gaubeca has little use for overbearing, under-informed doctors. She, like many of the people with diabetes profiled on these pages, has suffered from the "seven deadly sins" commonly committed by unenlightened doctors when treating people with diabetes:

1. guilt trips
2. suspicion
3. bullying and browbeating
4. ignoring deeper spiritual issues
5. fear mongering (also known as diabetic shock treatment)
6. patronizing
7. a failure to communicate

When she learned that I was working on a magazine proposal about the seven deadly sins, she rejoiced: "Yea! People with diabetes strike back!"

Gaubeca actually has "diabetes in her blood," but not in the usual sense of that term. Her great-grandfather, Francis Gano Benedict, was an early diabetes researcher who co-authored books with Elliott P. Joslin of the famous Joslin Clinic and Diabetes Center in Boston. At the time Benedict was working, before insulin was isolated in the 1920s, the average life span for people diagnosed with type 1, which was then called "serious diabetes," was about 14 months.

Having descended from a famous diabetes researcher, Gaubeca has spent much of her life researching the condition on her own terms, which are mostly spiritual in nature.

After growing up in Mexico City, Gaubeca got her B.A. degree in English literature and communications from Wilson College in Pennsylvania and began a lifelong quest for spiritual answers to her diabetic condition. As she told me, her spiritual quest was in response to the basic question many people with diabetes ask: "Good God, why are you picking on me?"

The answer she received, after years of soul-searching, was simple but powerful. "There's a good reason why I had diabetes," says Gaubeca. "Because it led me somewhere I didn't want to go."

In the process of going where she didn't want to go, she absorbed every spiritual philosophy from Tibetan Buddhism to atheistic existentialism; read anything from Thich Nhat Hahn and Pema Chodron to Stephen Covey and Harville Hendrix.

"I wasn't church-going," she says, "but I worshiped God in the cathedral of my heart."

Gaubeca was finding out much the same thing I did about the give and take of spirituality and diabetes. Diabetes inspired me to become more spiritual, which in turn inspired me to manage my diabetes better.

The Donut of Despair

One of her spiritual discoveries is what she calls, appropriately enough for a person with diabetes, the "Donut of Despair."

It goes like this. There are two circles in everyone's life. The inner circle is yourself and everything you can influence. The outer circle is those things you can't influence, even though they affect you. The more you ignore the inner circle and worry about the outer circle, the more life becomes a "Donut of

Despair." But the more you focus on the inner circle and accept the outer one as beyond your control, the more power you exercise over your life.

"It's absolutely true that my deeper spiritual awareness has given me more strength to handle the daily grind of managing diabetes," she concludes. "It's also helped me handle the rest of my life."

While handling the rest of her life, Gaubeca returned to school to earn her masters degree in public health, recently doing her two-month internship at a remote village in Guatemala as a health aid. The experience in the dangerous bush of Guatemala embodied Gaubeca's whole approach to life since taking her insulin dosages into her own hands as a teenager.

"It confirmed my own philosophy about being able to take care of myself and not being limited by diabetes," she says.

Pessimism Is Catching

She also tries to guide her fellow people with diabetes from munching on the "Donut of Despair."

While facilitating a support group for the American Diabetes Association, she noticed a significant difference in the health of the optimistic members, as opposed to the pessimists. In the group, where members range in age from 18 to 60, the optimists always appeared to have a healthy glow to match their upbeat attitude, while the pessimists always seemed to have physical complications.

"The worst part about the pessimists was when they'd monopolize the conversation," Gaubeca explains, "saying diabetes has been the cause of their ruin, and woe is me, and blah, blah, blah. That's when I found out pessimism is catching."

Practicing her own special brand of optimism, Gaubeca now spends much of her time doing spiritual exercises, including various kinds of meditation, designed to give her a mystical direction in life.

"Try not to be a tumbleweed," as she sums up her Eastern philosophy with a very Western metaphor.

In many ways, her own blood sugar has served as her lifelong guru.

"Perhaps I wouldn't have done any of this without diabetes," she says. "Now I realize that any time there's growth, there's pain. Suffering always makes us grow. When I look back at my life, I often say, 'Hmmm. That's the reason I got diabetes.'"

Jewett Pattee

Adult Onset Jock

"My church is on my bicycle," says Jewett Pattee about the activity that, along with running, helped resurrect him from the dead.

For the 79-year old pharmacist and phenom of Long Beach, California, he was converted to the spiritual practice of sport at the age of 50, when he was diagnosed with type 2 diabetes. At the time, by his own description, Pattee was a heavy smoker, a gentle tippler, a workaholic, and a walking pork chop. He tipped the scales at 50 pounds over his optimum weight, he religiously practiced the art of the couch potato on his days off, and his blood pressure had topped off at 220 over 110.

"I got to the point," Pattee says, "when I understood I had to do something. As a pharmacist,

I knew what was going to happen to my future if I allowed these degenerative conditions to work on me."

That fatal knowledge put a scare into him that sent him running for his life. Literally.

"I like life," Pattee says. "But the fear of death doesn't bother me. It's going down the tubes the bad way that scares me. I suddenly realized that people suffering from diabetes or other chronic illnesses have to make a big lifestyle change and stick with it if they want to keep a good quality of life."

What We've Been Put on This Earth to Rise Above

Perhaps Pattee understood the essence of what Rosy told Charlie in the classic John Huston film version of *The African Queen*: "Nature is what we've been put on this earth to rise above."

And rising above his nature is exactly what Jewett Pattee did. He heard the catchy tune being played by a seductive Pied Piper and, like me at that time, joined the running rat race.

That was 1972, when the running craze was just beginning to sweep the nation like an exercise in mass hysteria. Millions of people started reforming their health through running, which, as it turned out, was like flipping a coin. Yes, if the coin came up heads, it meant many long-term benefits, such as weight loss, aerobic fitness, stress reduction, and improved all-around health. But if the coin landed on tails, it brought on numerous aches and pains for people whose running form wasn't structurally sound, including destruction of major joints in the knees and hips. Pattee certainly got all the benefits of running, but eventually lost his coin toss.

His first goal was simply to stagger through an entire mile without stopping. That small victory inspired him to increase his mileage and gear up his speed. Within a year, he entered a Senior Olympics 1,500-meter race and finished third.

"I was losing weight, gaining energy, improving my confidence, and feeling better all around," he recalls about his new exercise regimen. "Then things got a little out of control."

In the ensuing years, as Pattee reached his middle fifties, he increased his training by quantum leaps and subsequently finished five competitive marathons. At last the impact of so much running caught up to his right hip, which he had to have replaced. But that didn't stop him either. Four marathons later, he had the same hip replaced again.

By the time Pattee was 62, he was clearly addicted to the athletic lifestyle that had transformed his health and made him a happier human being. But he was beginning to understand that running was no longer an option.

When Somebody Hits Me Over the Head

"When somebody hits me over the head with a club," Pattee says, "I eventually try to listen."

That's when he began cycling big time. What he has accomplished since then is unequaled by anyone in any of his various age groups over the years, or by few competitors of any age, for that matter. As an example, he has ridden on the four-man cycling teams that hold the records for both the grand masters and mixed masters 3,000-mile relay races across America, in which the team members take turns, one rider at a time, pedaling from California to Georgia.

His team's best time for that event, believe it or not, was about eight days and four hours. When Pattee was 75, his team of septuagenarians turned the trick in eight days, nine hours.

As he spins toward the age of 80, Pattee still rides and competes. His racing is co-sponsored by his healthcare provider (Secure Horizons of PacifiCare Health Systems) and the American Diabetes Association, and he is also his team's captain for the ADA's national cycling program, the Tour de Cure. In exchange for this support, he tries to raise awareness among people with diabetes that they can change their lifestyles, manage their diabetes, and totally reform their quality of living.

"Diabetes acted as the inspiration to overturn my life and revolutionize it," he says. "Diabetes has definitely helped me evolve as a human being. It's given me goals in life, kept my mental state sharp, made me personally happier, and given me a purpose I never dreamed of having: spreading the word that you have to control diabetes, rather than having it control you. It kicked me in the butt and got me going."

Michael Raymond

Adventures in Diabetes

Not all stories about courageous people with diabetes are happy ones. Some of them are about gaining acceptance, tolerance, and peace of mind in the face of terrible complications. One such story is that of Michael Raymond, a professor of English literature at Stetson University in De Land, Florida.

Diagnosed with type 1 diabetes in 1955, the 56-year-old Raymond has persevered through a series of setbacks (three open-heart surgeries, two amputations, impotence, and retinopathy) that he refers to, quite dryly, as "adventures."

Professor Raymond included many anecdotes about his diabetic adventures in a 1992 book, published by Noble Press of Chicago, titled *The Human Side of Diabetes: Beyond Doctors, Diets, and Drugs.*

"The basic philosophy of my book," he says, "is that 'We're not people with diabetes, we're human beings. I'm a person, not a pancreas with a body attached.'"

His great adventure began when he was diagnosed at the age of nine. As was common practice in those days, he was quickly shipped out to a famous diabetes clinic for a week of training, education, and orientation.

"Their whole strategy was to scare the hell out of me," Raymond says. "They told me I wouldn't live to be 21. That every soda I drank was a year off my life. They also stuck me in an adult ward and made sure there were diabetic patients who were blind, had amputations, had heart disease, and one who died while I was there. All that formed my vision of diabetes. They were trying to impress me, and they did."

Raymond also overheard his father telling a doctor, "Mike's life is over."

Young Mike Raymond's despair over diabetes soon turned to guilt. Like many people with diabetes before and after him, he felt as though each of his numerous urine tests was like failing a pop quiz in school. Largely as a result of his negative experiences with the medical community and the imprecise management techniques of the day, his maintenance was mediocre.

Still, through sheer force of will and determination, Raymond forged a productive life. He played many different sports. He earned his Ph.D. in 18th-century literature. He began a 30-year career teaching at Stetson. He married a loving woman, and together they had two fine boys.

This Suspicious Kind of Interrogation

In the early 1980s, Raymond even changed his bad attitude about diabetes. He was referred to the Diabetes Care Unit at Humana Lucerne Hospital in Orlando, Florida, where a number of nurses helped him resolve his pent-up anger, hostility, and guilt. Before then, as he says, he was used to the medical community grilling him with "this suspicious kind of interrogation" about his maintenance techniques. But here the staff treated him as a unique human being with a singular case of diabetes that had to be dealt with in his own way.

"Rather than beating myself up about how poorly I was doing with my management," recalls Raymond, "I learned to do the best I could, and leave it at that. I began treating each day as a new day, and tried to improve from there."

That attitude helped immensely when his series of crippling complications, as mentioned above, set in. Instead of regarding these painful experiences as some kind of Old Testament punishment, he now regards them as a kind of New Testament redemption.

Diabetes Has Made Me a Better Man

"There's no doubt that diabetes has made me a better man," he says, "and made me a better parent, a better husband, and certainly a better teacher."

Raymond cites his own ethical evolution as a human being as more proof of diabetes' positive effect on his life.

"When I was a kid," he remembers, "I was going to be a lawyer, just so I could crush people, and make money, and wield power. I wanted to strike back because diabetes made me feel so powerless. But look what I've evolved into as a person with diabetes. Now I'm a teacher."

Even his teaching approach has been formed by diabetes. One of his duties at Stetson—an exclusive school where, as Raymond says, the students are either "pre-law, pre-med, or pre-rich"—has historically been to teach what he calls the "anguish courses," the classes required in English lit. But instead of marching his students through the metrical footwork of iambic pentameter or the otherworldly rhyming of the metaphysical poets, he teaches them the human side of literature and how it reflects on their personal lives.

In the process, he's become the magnet for students troubled by medical conditions or emotional problems.

"I never would have taken the human approach," he says, "if I'd never had diabetes. Diabetes has made me a much stronger person both psychologically and spiritually. I'm much tougher and more resistant and more tolerant, mostly because I'm more accepting."

Jim Collins

Escape from the Sweatbox

Jim Collins describes type 1 diabetes as "living in a box." That's how he had felt for most of the last three decades, since being diagnosed with juvenile diabetes at the age of six. The box was both physical and mental, a "kind of void," as Collins says, where his blood sugar was often sucking away his energy, his mind was fog-bound, and he constantly lived with the feeling that something essential had been taken away from him. That "something essential" was his freedom.

"The box" had caused Collins to miss a lot of school as a child, mainly because he felt so lousy much of the time, and influenced him to lead a sedentary life, isolated from his siblings and devoid of playmates. He grew up, graduated from college, and became a professional sports photographer while suffering from that same sense of alienation. In truth, Collins had been living most of his life in a form of solitary confinement, imposed by his own hemoglobin level.

All *that* changed quite suddenly in 1998 while he was working as a volunteer staffer at a walkathon near his home in Newport Beach, California. That's when another volunteer asked him, "Why don't you run a marathon?"

Collins' response, fueled by his need for release from years of frustration, physical discomfort, and living in the box, was instantaneous.

"Yeah. Why not? I've gotta do something."

Team Diabetes

It was as if a key had been turned and a cell door opened in his mind. Suddenly, Jim Collins was set free.

That brief interaction led Collins to get involved with the American Diabetes Association's Team Diabetes running program, in which members meet on a regular basis, in places all over the world, for group distance runs. The comradery and support of Team Diabetes helped Collins discover he had a knack for running long distances. Within seven months of his first run, he had successfully completed a 13-mile half-marathon in San Diego and a full marathon in London, England. In the latter, he finished the 26-plus-mile race shortly after striding across London Bridge, in about seven hours.

Running was not only liberating for Collins, but addictive. Combined with the use of his new insulin pump, it stabilized his blood sugar, physically rejuvenated his body, lifted the mental fog shrouding his life, and gave him an overall feeling of euphoria. Of course, part of that effect can be attributed to the pain-killing endorphins continually released by long-distance running. But the whole running experience was mind-expanding for Collins.

"Now, when I look at the difference between the 'before' and 'after' pictures of myself, I can see where my newfound freedom has brought me," he says. "And I want to be there all the time. That makes me work harder at both running and blood-sugar management. I feel so much better, both mentally and physically."

Flat-lining the Nerve Tests

Running also produced a physical effect that rivals faith healing as a medical phenomenon. Before taking up running, Collins suffered from diabetic neuropathy in both feet, a condition that made his feet feel like wood, and his toes like they were all welded together.

"I had zero feeling in my feet," says Collins. "I was basically flat-lining the tests for nerve sensation."

But somehow running dramatically reduced the neuropathy, a positive reversal of fortune that amazed all of Collins' doctors. They could find no parallel event in medical records.

"Now, while I'm in training, my feet are basically normal," says Collins. "Or, at least, 90 percent of normal.

But when I was injured and couldn't train, the neuropathy came back with a vengeance. So, it's obvious I'm going to have to keep running for the rest of my life."

The life of a marathoner hasn't been all smooth running or fast striding for Collins. Shortly after his London marathon, he suffered a foot injury when the ground gave out on a dune where he was training. Then, in 2000, while he was running a half-marathon in Long Beach, California, he developed a stress fracture.

The down time, in both instances, convinced Collins that he's hooked for life.

"I had been a prisoner of my own diabetes," he says, "and now I'd made the Great Escape. I wasn't about to quit now."

Collins sees his running breakthrough as a miracle that is just as much spiritual in nature as physical. Before, when he was confined to the box, he was basically a pessimist who felt tired, run down, and depressed much of the time. But his accomplishments as a runner gave him a newfound power over his diabetes and his life.

"Now I realize that if I can do something as hard as a marathon," says Collins, "there isn't anything else standing in the way of what I want to achieve. Diabetes used to be in control of my life, and now I'm the one in control. I'm in the driver's seat now."

Joe Clifford

Dear Joe, We Hope You Don't Die

Joe Clifford still laughs at the get-well cards he received from all his sixth-grade classmates some 22 years ago. At the time he was hospitalized, "getting the full treatment" at a diabetes clinic during the week following his diagnosis. What Clifford finds so amusing about all the cards is that they represented the uncensored scuttlebutt related to his new case of diabetes.

As one card said, pulling no punches: "Dear Joe, we hope you don't die."

Clifford, who is now the editor of *Wentworth Magazine*, the alumni organ published by Wentworth Institute of Technology in Boston, appreciates the tactless spirit of these We-Hope-You-Don't-Die-Grams. He doesn't take his reality sugar-coated. No one is more

admiring of the truth, the whole truth, and nothing
but the truth than Joe Clifford.

The whole truth about blood sugar, according to
Joe Clifford, is that you can't do anybody any good by
feeling sorry for yourself.

"My attitude about diabetes," he says in straight
talk that belies his thoughtful demeanor, "is you ought
to check your self-pity at the door. I dislike self-pity in
others, and so I would be hypocritical if I indulged in it
myself. I think I've been very lucky in my life. I don't
think I have too much to complain about."

Crash Course in Diabetes

Clifford got his first crash course in diabetes in
1980. His sixth-grade basketball team was "awesome,"
as he recalls, and he was the star player. His team didn't
lose at all until the last game of the season, when he was
feeling incredibly sluggish. He spent the rest of that
weekend in a funk, trying to quench an unquenchable
thirst with gallons of Pepsi Cola. His symptoms
obviously worried his mother, who was seen with her
nose buried in a home medical guide, sometime before
telephoning his brother, who was then attending
medical school.

The following Tuesday, while young Joe was
walking home from school, his mother pulled up in her
car and told him to get in.

"We're going to the doctor," she said.

The family doctor, an old-fashioned gentleman
with a Marcus Welby bedside manner, broke the bad

news with what Clifford now calls "the comic book version" of diabetes.

"Joe, do you like candy bars?" the doctor asked.

"Sure," said Joe. He obviously liked Pepsi, too, because he had single-handedly kept the company in business for the last two weeks.

"Well," said the doctor, "you probably won't be eating a heck of a lot of sweets from now on."

Characteristically, Clifford took the blow in stride.

"Maybe this is the way I am in general," Clifford says, "but I was a little underwhelmed by the seriousness of the situation. For better or for worse, I'm from the Go-Into-Your-Room-And-Lick-Your-Wounds-And-Don't-Let-Anyone-See-You School of Life."

Clifford grew up managing his diabetes without any fanfare and refusing to use his condition as a crutch. All he asked was to be treated like everybody else. For instance, when he was a freshman pitcher on the Princeton University baseball team, he had an experience that still galls him. All candidates for the varsity team had to pass an early-season fitness test that included running a mile in under six minutes. On his first try at the mile, Clifford staggered across the finish line about 15 seconds above the cutoff point and began kicking himself for not starting practice in better shape.

Then an assistant coach pulled him aside and said, "You know, maybe we shouldn't have this test for you. It's probably hard for people with diabetes to run."

Clifford was both offended and embarrassed at being stereotyped this way, so he insisted on retaking the test, which he passed with all the other athletes.

"It didn't even occur to me there was any relationship between athletic training and diabetes," he says. "I find that sort of thinking totally offensive. You should never do that to yourself. Never treat yourself like a pariah."

A Shut-Up-and-Play-the-Game Kind of Guy

And he never has. Now Clifford has a wife and two young daughters, works at a challenging job, and goes about his existence with the firm conviction that he will never be scarred or marked by diabetes.

In that kind of uncompromising light, he looks at diabetes as a kind of pickup basketball game. Being a bonafide gym rat, Clifford has noticed two basic types of players in pickup games. One is the Alibi Ike style of competitor, those players who cover up for every mistake with a justification, make a rationalization for every bad pass, and call a foul after every missed shot.

"They're excuse-makers," says Clifford, "and self-pity is their currency."

Then there is the second type of competitor, those who simply shut up and play the game.

Clifford is a shut-up-and-play-the-game kind of guy, whether shooting hoops on the basketball court, or shooting insulin in the locker room.

He's the strong silent type in his spiritual life as well, which he sees as playing a crucial part in managing his diabetes. He describes himself as a "Cafeteria Catholic," meaning he reserves the right to pick one doctrine and pass on another, according to the dictates of his conscience.

"I'm not devout," he quips, "which by definition means I don't go to church as often as my mother."

But Clifford is metaphysical in the sense that he holds himself to a personal moral code and lives by a strict set of standards. And, with those standards in mind, he has observed a very close relationship between his own spirituality and diabetes.

"I would definitely say that, when I look at my diabetes through spiritual eyes," says Clifford, "it has helped me evolve as a human being. Diabetes teaches a certain discipline and responsibility about yourself, which in its spiritual essence is the way you should go through life."

In turn, his spiritual life has allowed him to get a better perspective on diabetes.

"If you're inclined to be spiritual, you're inclined to think long-term," he says. "Spiritual people aren't live-for-today people. By being conditioned spiritually to look toward the long-term, to think about consequences, whether they be ten years from now or after death, *that* tells a person with diabetes the right way to act and the right thing to do."

When asked what is the best long-term attitude for dealing with the daily task of diabetes management, Clifford shifts into editorial mode, mentally deleting all the dangling participles and typographical errors, cutting out all the purple prose to get at the uncluttered truth.

"Even-tempered acceptance," he says at last, "will always trump miserable resentment."

The Greatest Happiness

"The greatest happiness," said 18th-century French writer Madame de Staël, "is to transform one's feelings into action."

Now it's time for a practical course of action.

The rest of this book will demonstrate my own method for developing a holistic spiritual life, building a positive attitude, and taking control over diabetes.

Is taking control easy? Of course not. Nothing worthwhile is. But it is all part of the tempering process that all people with diabetes must go through to steel their character and activate their dreams.

"Character cannot be developed in ease and quiet," said writer and lecturer Helen Keller, who overcame her own blindness and deafness. "Only through experience of trial and suffering can the soul be strengthened, vision cleared, ambition inspired, and success achieved."

Such "trial and suffering" is the lasting gift of diabetes.

three

Zen and the Art
of Diabetes Maintenance

*A Spiritual
Guide for
People with
Diabetes*

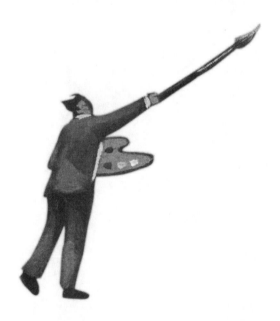

The Tao of Chaos

Seven Ways to Organize Your Soul

The more disorganized you are, the busier you appear to be. Call this observation the Tao of Chaos. Confusion, in other words, acts as a fine diversionary tactic. But, although the resulting flurry of activity might be good for fooling co-workers into overestimating your productivity, it's not very good for the spirit.

I have found that the more disorganized I am in spirit, the more my spirit is cluttered up with emotional busy work. The more disorganized my soul, the more my soul is paralyzed. I suspect the same might be true for you.

Part 3 of *Zen and the Art of Diabetes Maintenance* will give you a working model for beginning to organize your spirit and, with it, your health.

You have already seen in Part 1, through my own story, how diabetes can inspire a chain reaction of soul-searching, reevaluation, and spiritual improvement. You have seen in Part 2 how medical professionals have found that spiritual seeking creates numerous positive physical and emotional changes in people with diabetes, and how the spiritual inspiration triggered by diabetes has revolutionized the lives of many other people with diabetes.

Now it's time to put this spiritual energy to work for yourself.

"A new philosophy, a way of life, is not given for nothing," said Russian novelist Fyodor Dostoevski. "It has to be paid dearly for and only acquired with much patience and great effort."

It's true, you must pay for your new way of life, your control over diabetes, with much patience and great effort, but the process is a lot easier if it's an organized effort. In the following pages you will find the method I have developed to organize my own life into a kind of spiritual structure.

It would be absurd for me to pretend that any of the methodology I will present here is in any way original. Though spirituality involves discovering the innermost wisdom of your own self, the process of self-discovery is learned from a vast variety of outside sources. Some people find themselves in religion. Some in nature. Some in athletics. Others in artistic endeavor. Others in the wise counsel of those spiritual trekkers who have blazed the noble eightfold path before them.

In that context, I have begged, borrowed, and stolen my spiritual ideas from various cultures and many sources with more wisdom and knowledge and experience than myself.

"Transforming your mind takes time," said the Dalai Lama. "That isn't easy. It requires the repeated application of various techniques and taking time to familiarize yourself with the practices. It's a process of learning."

Through this process of learned practice, I have discovered something unique and immortal within my own soul. But I'm probably just like you. I'm no guru, and I'm no saint, and I'm certainly no master on matters of the spirit. Nevertheless, I am taking the lessons I have learned since being diagnosed with diabetes and formulating them into a new, more satisfying, more meaningful way of life.

My hope is that you can use my own model of spiritual practice as a very loose guideline for finding your own method. Certainly, you will discover that some of my suggestions are quite useful, and some are not very helpful for your particular situation. I am not in any way trying to perpetuate another kind of religious dogma to replace all those I've already rejected, and precisely because of their dogmatism.

The danger of any dogma is a kind of embalmed spirituality in which the prime motivation is a quest for perpetual life. As writer John Irving once observed, "Religion is just another kind of taxidermy."

I don't wish to be anybody's taxidermist, stitching some kind of make-believe immortality, made of sawdust and stuffing, into an empty skin.

As my Texas grandfather once told me in his gruff style: "Advice is no damn good to any old boy unless it makes a lick of sense."

Peace of mind is not an exact science, thank goodness. It is more of a very personal art form that you will have to perfect through your own trial and error.

Worshiping the Divine

I first learned the value of organized spiritual practice in a very relevant milieu: during my time as a visitor in the Abbey of New Clairvaux in northern California, while I was observing the measured, contemplative, prayerful, and deliberate lifestyle of monastic life.

At the abbey I soon realized I don't possess whatever faith, constancy, or discipline it takes to be a monk. And yet, I also sensed there is something deep and abiding that all of us, coming from whatever practice of religion or agnosticism we espouse, can take away from monastic practice. And by that I mean the systematic and sacred structure, the dogged methodology, monks use for worshiping the divine.

My eight-month exposure to the practice of Trappist monasticism has since imbued me with a systematic kind of grace, insight, and spiritual practice that is universal in its scope and all-embracing in its application. Now I understand how this metaphysical way of organizing my life, of slowing down my life, is every bit as powerful as the sweet chaos of hyperglycemia that makes me more busy than I ought to be, both emotionally and physically.

During my eventful stay at New Clairvaux, I met another accidental monk with a background similar to my own. His name was Brother Bob, a 90-year-old monastic who in his former career was a well-respected art director on many of Hollywood's most famous motion pictures of the 1930s and 1940s.

Even at the age of 90, he could still spin a mean yarn. Bob told me about wild Hollywood parties, including the drunken wrestling match between two famous directors that resulted in the destruction of his priceless Ming vase. He recalled the famous movie stars he had known—Mae West, for instance, with whom he traded frequent clever obscenities. Though Bob enjoyed his wild Hollywood partying, the lifestyle left him with a vague sense of dissatisfaction and lack of meaning. The antidote for this disenchanted state of mind turned out to be several miraculous incidents, which he detailed to me.

None of these events was more important than a religious locution in a redwood forest, in which a disembodied voice told him to give away everything he owned.

This last incident is what lead Brother Bob to the Trappists at the age of 60. Not being the sort of guy to ignore a mystical voice speaking to him in a redwood glade, he began searching far and wide to find a worthy recipient for his considerable family fortune. What he found as the object of his philanthropy was the monastery of New Clairvaux. Bob and the monastery's abbot quickly became fast friends. Soon thereafter, in that supernatural fashion that creates so many coincidences, Bob was also diagnosed with terminal cancer. Even after emergency surgery, he was given only hours to live.

It was at that critical moment when the abbot visited Bob in intensive care and gave him some far-reaching spiritual advice.

"Why don't you take vows, Bob, and become a monk?" the abbot told his friend.

"But I don't want to be a monk," said Bob. "I'm no more a monk than the man on the moon. I'm just not monk material."

"Well, heck," said the abbot. "You're going to die anyway. Why not die as a monk?"

A Man of Old-fashioned Integrity

So Bob took his vows. Then, in one of those miraculous developments that can never be explained by science or medicine or logic, Bob recovered from his cancer. In fact, he would survive for more than three more decades. And being a man of old-fashioned integrity, a man of his word, he abided by the vows he had made to the God in whom he believed. He lived out the rest of his life at New Clairvaux.

"That's how," as Brother Bob often groused, "God tricked me into becoming a monk."

Meanwhile, he discovered to his surprise that monastic life agreed with him. He thrived in the cloistered environment and intensive regimen of the monastery. He had somehow stumbled upon a medicine for the melancholy of life without direction and meaning. In the enduring practice of work, prayer, meditation, and sacred reading, and in the clockwork observance of the seven canonical hours, Brother Bob had found the satisfaction and faith that had been missing during his footloose years in Hollywood.

Now I look at Brother Bob's colorful story of the disease that changed his life as the perfect parallel for my own experiences with diabetes. He was a sugarman in monk's robes. Brother Bob's solution to his own spiritual search was the same as my own: a disciplined way of life in which the minute-by-minute observance of life's ambient elegance is the ultimate high.

Present-Moment Awareness

Monks and gurus and other spiritual seekers call this observance "present-moment awareness"—living totally in the here and now. I look at present-moment awareness as tantamount to taking a monastery with you wherever you go.

Eventually, after diabetes tricked me, much as Brother Bob had been tricked by his God, I would take what I learned at the abbey and transform it into my own kind of "canonical hours," the designated times during which monks stop whatever they are doing and dedicate themselves to brief periods of prayer and worship and present-moment awareness.

Spirituality finds strength in constancy. Whatever spiritual habits you adopt or adapt or invent, I recommend practicing them daily and with the same kind of routine and regularity that you monitor your blood sugar and diet. Your spiritual health is no less dependent on regularity than your physical health.

I have found the following spiritual habits helpful because each is like a path through a forest. Taking a well-marked trail through the woods is a pleasant, restful, invigorating, and life-celebrating experience that allows the hiker to observe the exquisite depth of nature.

At the time of this writing, there is one particular trail I've been walking almost daily, in a conservation area called Kent's Point near my current home on Cape Cod. The experience always combines both the solace of familiar landmarks and the thrill of knowing them in a new way each day. The fragrance of pine needles roasting in the sun; the sense of cricket-thrum and cicada-drone in the rough; the seabrine swelling toward Barley Neck; the shadow-light filtered through the leaves; the rush of feather-silk as goldfinches and waxwings and chickadees flick across my trail. These small events are so familiar, yet so miraculous, like a close brush with the supernatural each time I venture there.

Such daily inspirations result from a defined route of travel. But trying to penetrate a dark woods without any path to follow is another experience altogether. It is at once confusing, disturbing, and fearsome. You soon find yourself lost and disoriented. In that same way, a routine of regular spiritual exercise is the pathfinder for metaphysical trekking, and its routes are desire paths through the psyche.

As So Many Fools Prove Every Day

Nothing is foolproof, as so many fools prove every day. But the following set of spiritual activities works for me, even at my most foolish. These practices are the trails I have blazed for myself through the confusing, disturbing, and fearsome forest of existential questions that every person with diabetes must face about life. They are fine sedatives for my confusion.

My own spiritual way consists of seven basic practices that I try to carry out in timely fashion every day on my own journey toward discovery:

1. meditation
2. reading
3. solitude
4. exercise
5. awareness
6. prayer
7. clarification

These seven practices represent my own well-trod trail through the tangled underbrush of life and comprise the basic tenets of the spiritual guide I will detail in this section. I invite you to make this route your own, changing it to fit your own inclinations. Soon enough, as the Buddha said, you'll "become the Path" you are about to follow.

Telepathy of the Spirit
A Short Course in Meditation

I believe that meditation is absolutely indispensable for any person with diabetes. Not only is the regular practice of meditation beneficial for our medical and psychological well-being, but this healthful mental exercise produces a host of spiritual blessings.

Meditation, quite profoundly, is the telepathy of the spirit.

"Meditation is not a means to an end," said Indian philosopher Jiddu Krishnamurti. "It is both the means and the end."

Meditation can mean many things to many people. It can be based on concentration upon a mantra, a spiritual text, a chant such as an om, a bodily function such as breathing, or a mental image such as a bubble rising through a pond. Nobody can define the right kind of meditation for you.

But no matter what form a meditation takes, it is an activity that involves a "homecoming." By that I mean finding the person at the core of your very essence; meeting your own inner self, the one at the center of your being, who instinctively knows the answer to every dilemma in your life.

As spiritual teacher and author Lama Surya Das has said, "Meditation explores, investigates, unveils, and illumines what is hidden within and all around us."

Meditation also leads to self-seeking; coming home to your self while uniting your self with every other self. If you adopt nothing else from this book, at least begin to meditate. The benefits are boundless and the satisfactions are noticeable almost immediately. I like to call the practice my "transcendental medication."

The Forever Within Every Now

As the great Islamic prophet Muhammad said, "An hour's meditation is better than a year of adoration."

The first thing I perceived after beginning to meditate was the new way I looked at the world. Soon thereafter, I began to see the infinite in every leaf, in every bug, in every cloud. I began to sense the forever within every now. I began to know the cosmic intelligence within every sensation. I began to understand that the material world is but a symbol for something shimmering within its shadow. I began to sense the eternal weather within every cell.

Some might call this newfound awareness an incarnation of the traditional, religious God. I certainly don't dismiss that possibility, but I consider myself too limited in vision to make such a leap of faith. I never have been able to accept the anthropomorphic God, found in various holy books, who possesses all the earthbound foibles of wrath, vengeance, and intolerance that I dislike in human nature. I regard my own meditations as glimpses into some infinite spiritual force whose all-encompassing intelligence runs the universe and is totally beyond mortal comprehension.

I prefer the mystery of a godhood floating always beyond the veil of human perception. I prefer to accept the Buddha's careful approach to a supreme being. He refused to speculate about God, saying that the possibility of the creator's existence—what I like to call the "Big If" of human life—is a question we will never have the ability to answer for certain on this earth. So why worry about it?

"There ain't no answer," said Gertrude Stein. "There ain't going to be any answer. There never has been an answer. That's the answer."

Bulking Up the Muscle of Your Soul

The second thing I noticed after beginning to meditate was an increasing ability to concentrate. For, in essence, meditation is an exercise in concentration. And like any exercise, it progressively increases your ability to do whatever you are practicing. Meditation bulks up the muscle of your attention span and your soul.

The third, and perhaps most important, aspect of meditation is that through some automatic process within this spiritual exercise, I have gradually come to know myself better. I understand my motivations more thoroughly, I lie to myself less often, I act more at home with my feelings, and I feel more at peace with my place in the universe. In every way, meditation has served as a homecoming after many years of wandering in the wilderness of my misconceptions.

The list of other benefits reads like a litany of self-improvement. Meditation:

- provides moral direction and clarity in our lives
- gives us more confidence in our own inner strength
- makes us feel more grounded and secure
- makes us more conscious of life's meaning
- improves our mental acuity
- increases our sense of universal and personal love
- makes life seem more organized and sensible
- serves as a kind of instinctive psychotherapy, but without the self-pity
- gives us more intense humility
- makes our perceptions more insightful
- improves our mental and physical health as people with diabetes

The Meditative Biorhythm

I have found, going against all advice on this matter, that the best time for my own mediation is around noon, right after finishing my writing for the day. Some meditation guides, by contrast, recommend meditating twice a day, usually before breakfast in the mornings and before dinner in the evenings, and spending a total of 20 minutes to a half-hour at each meditation. Others suggest variations on this theme. But, somehow and for some reason I can't explain, I seem to flourish in the practice of one longer noontide meditation. You should experiment with different times and durations to find your own meditative biorhythm.

Thus, I spend about an hour meditating in a quiet place by concentrating on a mantra that I mentally repeat over and over to myself. The object is to focus on this mantra, and nothing else. When my mind wanders, as it will soon do, I simply bring my concentration back to my mantra in a gentle and nonjudgmental way. I might not even realize I've lost my focus on the mantra for some time. A few seconds, or even minutes, might pass, when suddenly I find myself thinking about baseball trades, or what I'll cook for dinner, or some writing I've been working on. After I become aware of my wandering mind, I don't beat myself up. I simply move my thoughts in a gentle way back to the mantra. It's something like re-grooving the needle on a record that's stuck.

The key is not to berate oneself for lack of discipline. Everyone's mind wanders, even the saints, holy people, and mystics who invented and practiced meditation during the past few thousand years. Meditation wouldn't be worthwhile unless focus were difficult. To paraphrase one Christian hermit, the mind in meditation is like an untrained stallion that will never be fully broken.

There are many mantras in use, or you can make up one that means something special to you. For example, I am currently using the mantra "sugarman" for obvious reasons. "Diabetes" would make another fine mantra.

As simple as this exercise in concentration sounds, it is astronomically difficult. Try lifting a small barbell over and over for 60 minutes straight and see how monumental a feat it becomes. The same is true of meditation. That is the utter beauty, the utter simplicity, and the utter impossibility of it. But soon your sense of well-being will transcend the difficulty of the task.

Sometimes, I vary this routine by using a meditation called breath counting, in which I focus my attention on counting my breaths, in-and-out, in-and-out, from one to ten. I concentrate only on the breath count and the physical sensations of my own breathing. Nothing else. Then I repeat the process, counting my own breaths from one to ten, over and over, for a span of about 20 minutes.

The Universe in a Raisin

Television commentator Bill Moyers, in his 1993 book *Healing the Mind*, wrote about a group meditation run by Jon Kabat-Zinn, a molecular biologist, medical professor, and founder of the stress reduction clinic at the Massachusetts Medical Center. The scene, as described by Moyers, found 25 "everyday, garden-variety Americans" sitting in a circle, some on the floor, others in folding chairs, their eyes closed, as they performed the sacred rite of . . .

Eating raisins.

"Slowly," Kabat-Zinn said from the center of this circle of raisin eaters. "Lift one raisin slowly to your mouth. Chew it very slowly. Observe your arm lifting the raisin. Think about how your hand is holding it. Now put it in your mouth and think about how it feels there."

And so the meditation continued, concentrating on the taste of the raisin, its effects on their salivary glands, the feel of the fruit on their tongues, its stickiness in their teeth.

The technique was as old as meditation itself, as common as breathing. Take some mundane, everyday act and give it total concentration. See it in every possible light, observe it with every possible sense, appreciate it with every possible feeling.

"They're really meditating," Kabat-Zinn later told Moyers. "Only we don't call it that. The word meditation tends to evoke raised eyebrows and thoughts about mysticism and hocus-pocus . . . So we call it 'stress reduction.'"

Once a week for eight weeks, Kabat-Zinn took groups of hurting and stressed-out patients through mindfulness practices such as the raisin meditation, yoga exercises, and body scanning (a concentration method for relieving pain). At the time of Moyers' book, more than 6,000 people had taken the stress-reduction program and 72 percent of them reported long-term moderate to significant improvements, both physical and psychological, in the various kinds of pain- and stress-related symptoms that had brought them to the clinic.

"The results suggest to me that people may be changing on a much more profound level over the course of these eight weeks than simply having the headaches disappear, or living with their back pain better, or watching their blood pressure go down," said Kabat-Zinn. "They may be undergoing some sort of rotation in consciousness that allows them to have a different relationship with their body and with their mental activities, as with the outside world."

As I have said, there are numerous ways to meditate, and every person must find the right form for himself or herself. But Kabat-Zinn had put his finger on a key component of every meditation: "a rotation in consciousness" that produces a profound change in the meditator's relationship to his or her own body, mind, and the world in general.

An in-depth discussion on meditation is the stuff of an entire book, or even the content of a whole lifetime. So I recommend consulting the titles on meditation in your library. Why not check out a few books on meditation and test some of the various forms before deciding on your own preference? In many ways, the process is like trying out a number of exercise routines to see which of them is best for your own lifestyle, talents, and predispositions.

I like to think of meditation as a "Doppler shift." Dutch physicist Christian Doppler discovered that as an observer moves away from the source of a light or sound wave, the measured frequency of that wave changes quite significantly. Likewise, meditation causes us to move away from the source of our own self-delusion, thus creating a Doppler shift in how we observe and measure the quality of life.

My own Doppler shift has affected practically everything I perceive, everything I do, and everything I am.

"Each soul must meet the morning sun, the new, sweet earth, and the Great Silence alone!" said the 20th-century Sioux writer and physician Ohiyesa.

Meditation is the mind's way of greeting the soul's Great Silence.

Book of the World
Suggestions for Spiritual Reading

edieval monks looked at creation as a *liber mundi*, a book of the world, where, as psychologist and spiritual writer Thomas Moore said, "They could read eternal truths and divine mysteries." My own *liber mundi* is the vast body of work written throughout history by seekers of wisdom and truth.

Reading, in one way or another, makes good sense out of a seemingly unruly universe. For, certainly, the chaotic nature of being is one of the overwhelming sensations that bombards anyone newly diagnosed with diabetes. Reading well-formed thoughts written by deep thinkers is one tried and true means of getting a reeling world under control.

As a person trying to improve my spiritual acuity in the face of diabetes, I have found spiritual reading absolutely indispensable. This is a golden age for spiritual literature. At no time in the history of human civilization has there been so much writing available to so many spiritual pilgrims. In a world in which there are far too few gurus and saints to go around, the publishing industry has transformed libraries into Tibetan monasteries, yoga centers, desert hermitages, and religious pulpits.

Just as medical breakthroughs surrounding diabetes make this the best time in history to be a person with diabetes, so the proliferation of spiritual writing makes this the best time in history for a person with diabetes to find meaning.

Solace Among the Book Stacks

Soon after I was diagnosed with diabetes, I did pretty much what you were doing when you picked up this book. I went looking for solace among the book stacks. Unfortunately, I couldn't locate any books akin to *Zen and the Art of Diabetes Maintenance* that give people with diabetes their own personal spiritual guide for treating their own medical condition and improving their own human condition. That paucity of writing on the spiritual implications of diabetes, as you have seen, was one major reason why I decided to write this book. But I did find plenty of spiritual material that, by implication, I could apply to my diabetes.

I have discovered that it doesn't take a lot of reading to bring me solace every day. In fact, sometimes a few paragraphs or pages or verses can fill me with enough food for thought to keep me digesting for the rest of the day.

"Make your own bible," said Ralph Waldo Emerson. "Select and collect all the words and sentences that in all your reading have been to you like the blast of triumph out of Shakespeare, Seneca, Moses, John, and Paul."

The Far-flung Territory

What kind of books am I talking about as food for my thoughts? Spiritual guides. Philosophical tracts. Books of meditations. Novels with metaphysical implications. Poetry. Natural History. Even science fiction. Anything that makes me think about the profound mysteries of the universe. This is the far-flung territory of reading that gives me comfort and consolation.

For example, let me give you a list of the readings on my shelf right now:

- *The Art of Loving* by Erich Fromm
- *A Confederacy of Dunces* by John Kennedy Toole
- *Care of the Soul* (A Guide for Cultivating Depth and Sacredness in Everyday Living) by Thomas Moore
- *The Art of Happiness* (A Handbook for Living) by His Holiness the Dalai Lama and Howard C. Cutler, M.D.

- *Ape and Essence* by Aldous Huxley
- *A Little Course in Dreams* by Robert Bosnak
- *Diabetes and Hypoglycemia: How You Can Benefit from Diet, Vitamins, Minerals, Herbs, Exercise and Other Natural Methods* by Michael T. Murray, N.D.
- *West with the Night* by Beryl Markham
- *The Heat Is On* (the Climate Crisis, the Coverup, the Prescription) by Ross Gelbspan
- *Leaves of Grass* by Walt Whitman
- *The Best Spiritual Writing of 1998* edited by Philip Zaleski
- *Desolation Angels* by Jack Kerouac
- *No Nature* by Gary Snyder
- *Awakening to the Sacred* by Lama Surya Das
- *The Poisonwood Bible* by Barbara Kingsolver

Buffeted by the Sweet Storm

It often strikes me that soulful writing is the kind of sacred communication, much like the religious locutions perceived by Brother Bob in his redwood copse, that requires both a voice to speak the truth and a person to hear it.

I never forget, when I open a new book, that the conjunction of coincidence, fate, and synchronicity that caused me to pick up this reading is much like the fateful interactions we have with each person we meet each day. There often seems to be some life-changing message to be found there, if only we had the vision to see it; if only we had the extra senses to hear the trees falling in the forests, needed to form the books we read.

Life, in a very real way, is a scavenger hunt for all the hidden meanings found in everyday activities. Accordingly, reading is the distiller of all hidden meanings everywhere.

The Grand Silence

Spending Time in Solitude Each Day

And now for a brief moment of silence. We can dedicate this moment to the peace and quiet that seems to be the ultimate victim of a modern lifestyle based on noise, constant access to radio or TV, a manic obsession with computers and cell phones, and the worship of hyperactivity.

Society in the frontier of the new millennium seems to treat solitude and silence as enemies of the state. Big Brother need not be watching if we always have enough din and disturbance to distract us.

What is behind this deep suspicion of solitude and whatever stillness resides within it? Wherever we go, we seek noise. Boom boxes blare. Jets roar. A disembodied mechanical voice informs us that "You've got mail." Blasting stereos turn automobiles into quaking bass drums. Televisions rave. Buzz saws howl. Car horns and squealing brakes and revving motors and howling sirens punctuate our every move. Drivers—terrified of losing touch with what?—even attach themselves in umbilical fashion to their squawking telephones.

Racket has become the substitute for thought, and cacophony the soundtrack for existence.

A Libido for Noise

Many of us seem intent on creating a world in which we never have to face "The Sounds of Silence," as Simon and Garfunkel so poetically expressed the extrasensory components of stillness. Could the reason behind our libido for noise be some deep-seated fear of self-knowledge, which we have effectively imprisoned within a wall of sound?

Certainly, such a realization has occurred to millions of spiritual sojourners over the centuries when they sought out the stillness of deserts and caves and mountain retreats and monasteries and nunneries and cloisters, shutting out the world of noise distracting them from matters of the spirit. Trappists, for example, lead their daily life in the regular observance of silence, refraining from speaking for long periods of time. Religious communities from various denominations call this practice the grand, or the noble, silence.

Taking my cue from their example and from many books advising silence as a spiritual practice, I try to re-create a slice of the silent life, a moment of the grand silence, a breath of the noble silence, every day.

"The point of passing time in silence," said Professor Phyllis D. Rose of Wesleyan University in an essay from the *Atlantic Monthly* (which was included in Philip Zaleski's fine anthology *The Best Spiritual Writing of 1998*), "is to strip yourself bare, to discover what is essential and true."

A Separate Peace

All should seek their solitude in their own ways. I personally prefer sitting on a quiet bench located in the woods, or overlooking a beautiful viewpoint, or down by the water's edge.

Simplicity is the key element in my silence. Sometimes I *simply* meditate. Sometimes I *simply* marvel at the staggering complexity of nature. Sometimes I *simply* contemplate the state of my life in the soothing atmosphere of a separate peace. Sometimes I *simply* listen to the breeze winnowing through the leaves, or water lapping against the sand, or birdsong playing through the woods; not noiselessness, strictly speaking, I know, but still a grand silence of a kind, a noble solitude of sorts. A quiet simplicity.

"We can be educated by nature," wrote Thomas Moore, "becoming persons of broad vision and subtle values. In nature we can find our place, our identity, and our affections."

Solitude and silence, I believe, serve several practical purposes for a person with diabetes on a spiritual mission. People with diabetes especially need the kind of respite that slows down their metabolism and lessens the stresses and strains of daily life, just as we have learned from the advice of medical experts in Part 2 of this book.

As a good example, during one very stressful period of my life, just after a knee operation, my fasting blood-sugar readings each morning averaged more than 110. Three months later, when I reached an extremely peaceful and satisfying period, my morning blood-sugar readings averaged around 90. I believe your own blood-sugar journal will show the same moderating pattern of blood sugar as stress is relieved.

Periods of silence serve to create a sort of demilitarized zone between us and our worries. A firebreak between our souls and the heat of a frenzied life.

The Dowsers of True Identity

Silence, like meditation, also tends to slow down the chatter of our thoughts, which often race out of control without us even being aware. The chaos of runaway thoughts is one of the most destructive forces there is for our innermost lives. Mental hyperactivity keeps a whole hidden world of understanding and wonder at bay.

As the great novelist Franz Kafka expressed the benefits of silence: "You need not leave your room. Remain sitting at your table and listen. You need not even listen, simply wait. You need not even wait, just learn to become quiet, and still, and solitary. The world will freely offer itself to you to be unmasked. It has no choice; it will roll in ecstacy at your feet."

Most of all, solitude and silence act as the dowsers of true identity, working like the sap in a divining rod to search out the subterranean depths of soul, self, and essence. And like divining, this powerful practice of silence operates through a mysterious strength, a muscular biochemistry, that none of us can explain.

"Nature and God—I neither knew," wrote Emily Dickinson. "Yet both so well knew me they startled, like Executors of My identity."

A Nervous Breakdown of Biblical Proportions

I found out about the healing power of silence first-hand when I retreated to the cloister of New Clairvaux while I was suffering from my nervous breakdown of biblical proportions, mentioned earlier. The noise of my anxieties and fears had made me literally non-functional. But gradually the silence and peace and meditation of the monastery began to work its magic on my soul. Since discovering the elixir of quietude at that Trappist monastery, and taking it with me wherever I went, I have never again suffered from such intense emotional pain and agony.

I used to be the daring young man on the flying trapeze, soaring from one illusion to the next in my quixotic way. But, after learning of my diabetes in 1996, silence would act like a safety net protecting me from acts of unrelenting danger, stress, and noise. Once I discovered solitude, I knew I could drop into this waiting embrace anytime I needed and give myself to the cat's-cradle of silence, holding me in its steady and calming grip.

Exercises in Fertility

The Spirituality of Sport

I know that some of my friends with diabetes regard exercise as more of a torture test than a spiritual practice. But I look at exercise as the oxen that pulls the plow of my spirit. For me, at least, exercise guarantees that I reap what I sow.

Exercise is absolutely necessary for the physical well-being of a person with diabetes. Here I want to add *spiritual* well-being to the benefits of exercise. Just as a well-conceived exercise regimen develops the fitness of all those bodily systems at risk from diabetes, so it flexes and strengthens and hardens and tones and fortifies the tissues of the soul.

My more skeptical friends, who have witnessed my behavior throughout what I often refer to as my "hyper-extended youth," would probably argue that my life-long love affair with exercise has less to do with spiritual seeking than with the pain-killing and mind-altering endorphins secreted during exertion. They're partially right.

I suspect that the morphine-like effects of endorphins are life's best natural high and make each day's exercise something like the vision quests of Native Americans and the peyote-driven enlightenment of Don Juan. What better way to explore the supernatural depths of the soul than by dosing oneself with the natural, safe, and beneficial narcotic of an exercise routine?

The Psychedelic Blessings of Exercise

Just to give you one good example of the psychedelic blessings of exercise, take its inspirational effect. Since my days as a penniless young poet composing obscure verses in the mist-shrouded landscape of Vancouver Island, I have always noticed the sublime role my daily running regime played in my writing. It was an odd day, for sure, when some form of creative idea or literary enlightenment or poetic insight didn't occur to me while I was striding through the vapor-locked hills of British Columbia.

That pattern of exercise-induced brainstorming has continued to this day: 30 years of creative energy, divided into thousands of workouts that have fueled my whole writing career. How do such workouts feel? Every serious athlete knows about the phenomenon of second wind. Any run usually feels miserable at first, with the runner experiencing heavy legs, hard breathing, and sore muscles. Then, a few minutes into the workout, you can sense all your veins and arteries opening up, as your lungs pump soothing oxygen to all your tissues. The other thing that opens up is your mind. At that point, your heavy legs grow springy, your pace seems smoother and more at ease with the earth, your body turns feathery and aerodynamic. Not long after that, the pain-killing endorphins begin bathing your system, accompanied by airy new thoughts and brilliant brain waves.

It wasn't by accident that many years ago, while working for a newspaper in Nova Scotia, I named a comical column I wrote "Second Wind." The piece contained all the whimsical and off-the-wall ideas I conjured up each day on my runs, while I was operating under the influence of second wind. In that same vein, many of the images, metaphors, and allusions that go into my articles, books, and poems have been spin-doctored by running and its mind-altering substances.

If my own experience as a wild-eyed runner plumbing the depths of the creative mind is not proof enough of sport's blessings, then I urge you to try endorphins yourself. All you have to lose is your distaste for exercise. Believe me, the experience is addicting, as I can testify with my own dirty little running habit.

A Tiny, Life-enhancing Pilgrimage

Of course, running isn't for everyone. But almost every person with diabetes can find a kind of exercise and an amount of activity right for himself or herself. As I have grown older and found myself more injury prone, I have learned to do with my exercise what stock-market gurus suggest for investing. Diversify.

Yes, I still love to run, but there are also many other kinds of exercise that keep me in glowing touch with my endorphins. Gardening, biking, basketball, tennis, house work, hiking, swimming, Nautilus training: These are all pursuits I have known and loved. There is a wide diversity of these athletic venues waiting for you to enjoy as well.

As I am writing this section of the book, during summertime on Cape Cod, I am also developing a new exercise routine that combines several of the spiritual practices prescribed on these pages. It is a regimen that each day is very much like taking a tiny, life-enhancing pilgrimage.

Starting from our cabin overlooking Arey's Pond, I hike the back road that winds in and out of the pretty woods and tiny supernatural mysteries surrounding Arey's Pond and Mayflower Point.

The sights I notice along the road are all astounding, and, for those of us who look beyond the apparent reality, each poses a mystery in itself. As I walk, I ask myself the hidden meaning behind each peculiar phenomenon I sense: the mystique of the prophetic cormorant always perched upon the same Styrofoam float; the enigmatic signboard for Carbo's Socratic Sailing School ("We teach questions, not answers"); the natural puzzle of the swans that always return to Arey's Pond late each summer; the mystery of the bell that rings from nowhere; and the secret behind the wrought-iron poodle wearing a tutu.

I take much pleasure in these cosmic brain teasers, posed by the interstellar trickster himself and washed up on these sandy shores by the daily ebb and flow of life.

On my walk, I contemplate the existential riddles raised by my surroundings, or perhaps I simply zone out. Walking, as you might have discovered for yourself, provides a meditative rhythm that allows one to lose oneself in what I call the "multiple climax of moments," each a flashpoint of ecstacy, moment by moment, that epitomizes what living should be all about.

My walk takes me rambling over hill and dale for about a mile and a half, at which point I reach a pretty pond called Crystal Lake, with a small swimming beach and a sparkling expanse of open water. Here I strip down to my bathing suit and do a half-hour swim into the middle of the lake and back.

As I stroke, I enjoy the soul-wetness of water caressing my skin and the thrill of my bodily engine firing on all cylinders. I welcome the narcotic secretions flowing from within and bathing my thoughts with inspiration.

Glimpsing My Own Soul

When I reach the center of Crystal Lake, I always stop for a few minutes to languish like a water strider on the surface and enjoy the willowy nature of the universe surrounding me. I watch the shape-shifting clouds forming their own silvery ink-blot test in the sky, and stare into the aqua-marine depths of the pond, an experience not unlike glimpsing my own subconscious.

Later, after drying myself off, I continue my pilgrimage. About a half-mile from Crystal Lake is the conservation area I mentioned earlier in this book, Kent's Point, a compact little Shangri La of woodlands, hiking trails, bayside viewpoints, and arresting enlightenment. Here I continue my rhythmic striding, toe-heel, toe-heel, toe-heel, relishing the syncopation of my own limbs working together in a conjunction of biochemical reactions, electrical impulses, mental stimuli, and muscular coordinations.

These interactions amount to proof positive that something quite extraordinary and mystical is at work, running the universe.

The point of Kent's Point is the point itself, a spot overlooking Barley Neck and, in the distance, Little Pleasant Bay. Here a bench is located in a lovely spot, where the shining currents of Barley Neck can be enjoyed through the cottonwood, oak, and pine trees. Even the metal inscription on the bench is a telltale indication of the holiness to be found there. The small plaque is a memorial for someone called Everett Mark Hafner: "His soul is at peace in this beloved place."

Here I like to spend 30 to 45 minutes in repose, silence, and meditation, a religious experience which seems to be blessed by the prevailing breezes of Kent's Point whispering through the treetops like a Gregorian choir, its humors echoing inside the leafy cathedral of these woods.

Reality Transubstantiated Into a Stained-glass Window

I've noticed an interesting phenomenon that seems to happen quite often during my sacred rite at Kent's Point, how the leaves tend to take on an external aura, and how the light here begins to soak everything with an otherworldly translucence, as if reality has been transubstantiated into a stained-glass window. Perhaps such perception is only my mind playing tricks on itself. Or perhaps the world of materiality is showing its true colors, characterized by those celestial hues hiding within every solid-state thing.

Whatever their source, I firmly believe that the visions of my exercising are a physical manifestation of my own inner life. Likewise, I feel certain that exercise is both a physical and spiritual habit that has lasting rewards for any person with diabetes. And, finally, I have faith that my physical discipline is part and parcel of the spiritual conditioning that the Dalai Lama prescribes for the pursuit of happiness.

"So, engaging in training or a method of bringing about inner discipline within one's mind is the essence of a religious life," he has said, "an inner discipline that has the purpose of cultivating positive mental states."

Nature Being Aware of Itself
The Benefits of Self-awareness

Joining the rank of the devoutly religious involves the regular practice of experiencing the mystical, acknowledging the impenetrable, and exploring the self. It involves what might be summed up in one term—"self-awareness."

Self-awareness, in fact, is humanity's most precious gift, a higher function that essentially separates humans from the remainder of earth's creatures. We are nature being aware of itself, to paraphrase a quote from Erich Fromm, mentioned earlier on these pages.

Many psychoanalysts such as Fromm practice a form of self-awareness that is highly logical, based on the scientific approach to psychology pioneered by Sigmund Freud and carried on by Carl Jung and many other researchers studying human mental disorders. The awareness I mean here is more soul-searching, and less deductive, in character. I look at such awareness as the difference between how Sigmund Freud and Francis of Assisi might have looked at the world: the first by applying all the concentrated power of his deductive reasoning; the second by focusing the immense brightness of his intuitive instinct.

One at a Time and Second by Second

And what, you might well ask, are we to become aware of? The answer is every thing; but only one at a time, and always second by second.

Coming from my own background of self-deception and negativity, I need to aim my awareness on the inner workings of my daily behavior; on the negative reactions I've developed over the course of my life as response to the rigors, stresses, and troubles that every person encounters.

Like most people I know, I have developed a set of negative conditioned reflexes to handle my daily problems. Most of these reflexes are not only ineffectual, dysfunctional, and anxiety-producing when employed against life's trials and tribulations, but they are based on misconceptions.

As one illustration, when some stranger says something rude and insensitive to me, I tend to take it personally. But by taking a moment to practice awareness, by aiming an intuitive spotlight on this kind of interaction, I usually realize how this person, rude or not, actually means me no harm. Maybe he or she had a fight with a spouse, or was ostracized by a boss, or suffered a death in the family. Perhaps, for a person in pain, making uncivil remarks becomes more or less unconscious, like killing a fly with a swatter. Who knows? Maybe such rudeness is totally unintentional, akin to jostling a stranger by accident in a crowded subway car.

A Course Through the Bloodlines of Our Ancestors

This is only one example of the numerous small hurts that self-awareness can cure each day. Another is my own intolerance.

My biggest fault is an overly critical attitude. I'm far too judgmental. This tendency probably comes from a childhood living with the raging paranoia of my stepfather, who himself was a victim of the bad attitudes and suspicious love of his mother. Most hurtfulness and intolerance can be traced, much like some diabetes, in a course through the bloodlines of our ancestors.

But that doesn't mean we have to let such wrongful logic make us unhappy too, like a bad seed being passed by genetic code from generation to generation.

The antidote for self-delusion is self-awareness. And the exercise of self-awareness is as simple as it is difficult. Each time you find yourself engaging in any conditioned reflex that triggers negative emotions in yourself, that fills you with a vague sense of unhappiness and discontent, merely stop and take stock. Consider what has just happened. Understand your own negative response. Look at the unadulterated reality of the situation. Let yourself envision a more fitting response. Then, let the truth, like a cascade of holy water, wash over you.

By the dogged practice of self-awareness all the time, you will make yourself into a happier, more fulfilled human being. Negative conditioning will gradually disappear, and so will many of your fears, anxieties, angers, delusions, and annoyances. Your life will not only simplify itself, but your day-to-day relationships will become much more fruitful and life-enhancing.

Sober Rumination in a Soulful Place

"The most beautiful emotion we can experience is the mystical," said Albert Einstein. "It is the power of all true art and science. To know what is impenetrable to us really exists, manifesting itself as the highest wisdom and the most radiant beauty, this knowledge, this feeling, is at the center of true religiousness. In this sense, and in this sense only, I belong to the rank of the devoutly religious."

Another exercise in awareness has to do with what Einstein called the "impenetrable" nature of the mystic. Glorying in life's mystery is a painless and mind-expanding practice that I try to do regularly throughout my day. It involves the humble task of taking a break.

Ever so often, whenever the mood strikes me, I stop my writing or whatever else I'm doing and enjoy a few minutes of sober rumination in a soulful place. Here, in this cottage where I am writing, I merely step out the front door and sit on our fieldstone steps. I am suddenly surrounded by woods and sky and the quiet brilliance of Arey's Pond shining through the trees.

Then I enjoy the weather, be it moody or fair, or inhale the fragrance of fresh-mown grass, or take a few deep swills of the salty sea breeze, or regard the everyday majesty of nature and all its secret manifestations. Awareness is its own reward, and the reward in turn is deeper awareness.

With a little imagination, I'm certain you can arrive at your own methods of awareness. For, to be sure, a person with diabetes exercising the rites of newfound spirituality has much to be aware of. As I have found, diabetes sweetens us with the awareness of a whole new world opening up. And what that world inspires is living every day as though it were the last. Being aware of every minute as though it were the final.

Blood sugar is a signal, sent from second to second by our cells, that life is short.

"Just to be is a blessing," said Rabbi Abraham Hershel. "Just to live is holy."

The Common Language
of the Soul
Prayer and the "Big If"

Just as "You'll never find an atheist in a foxhole," you probably won't find many people with diabetes who don't pray; even, like me, when they don't know exactly to whom or what they are praying. If there is anything I do which can be described as an act of blind faith, prayer fits that bill.

It is with some amount of deep concern that I even use the term "prayer" to describe the acts of petition I regularly perform as a person with diabetes searching for enlightenment. Over the centuries, the meaning of prayer has been abused and misused almost as much as the name of God, which has been invoked to rationalize every kind of obscenity, from war to hatred to prejudice to genocide.

As a person who went through nine years of Catholic school, I was taught that prayer was basically a rigid formula of words I didn't understand for obtaining blessings I couldn't comprehend.

As just one example, for years as a child I believed God's name was Hal. The evidence for this matter of faith was contained right in the Lord's Prayer. "Our father, who art in heaven," I recited with deep feeling every day, "*Hal* will be thy name."

That childhood misunderstanding took on an additional life of its own for me years later, when I first attended "2001: A Space Odyssey" and discovered that the computer representing the god figure was named Hal. Here, in this coincidence, was the poetic justice that embodied the mechanical kind of God and the encoded kind of prayer I learned as a kid.

The Mindless Greed of Prayer

Let's face the fact. The mindless greed of prayer as used in many modern religions has become a cliche. I have to wince, for example, every time I see a baseball player crossing himself before he steps into the batter's box or a team gathered in prayer before a game. In a world full of environmental catastrophe, war, torture, starvation, disease, pain, and nuclear weapons, prayer should not be something wasted on our day-to-day pettiness, trifles, or games.

All that said, there is still something sacred and universal about the use of prayer for obtaining our heartfelt desires. Several years ago, many people laughed when a group of Buddhist monks, clad in their traditional orange robes, gathered beside Boston Harbor to pray for its environmental recovery from centuries of pollution. That act, to me, is what real prayer is all about: humbly changing the universe through sheer force of will and reverence.

My childhood friend, Al Hall, who now works as a carpenter on Cape Cod, is a fallen-away Catholic like myself, a response to being drilled by *The Baltimore Catechism* in dogma that possessed all the soul of a traffic citation.

Even so, Al rediscovered prayer in his mid-life after his sister gave him a statue of St. Jude, the Patron Saint of Lost Causes. He found through a process of careful observance that if he wrote a note about something that was very important to him, and slipped it under the plaster statue, his wish seemed to come true. Al doesn't know exactly why this cause and effect takes place, nor what kind of mystical force is behind it, but he regards the process with all due reference.

"Why it happens, I don't ask," Al told me. "But I always approach the act with respect."

"Prayer, like meditation, is a complex concept with multilevel meanings from age to age, religion to religion, and culture to culture," wrote Lama Surya Das. "The common theme in all traditions, however, revolves around the natural human wish to open our hearts and communicate with the sacred principle, a higher power, or divine source. Whatever language we may use, prayer is the common language of the soul."

St. Augustine said all that and more when he made the following prayer: "Whisper in my heart, tell me you are there."

A Quantum Leap into Outer Space

Deepak Chopra, who is a synthesizer of much spiritual, philosophical, and scientific thought, explains prayer (though Dr. Chopra doesn't call it *that*) as a kind of transcendental access to the quantum field of physics, in which matter and energy are connected in an infinite ecosystem that can be influenced by our awareness, our intention, and our desire.

In other words, "prayer" is a form of mind over matter (though Dr. Chopra might not use *that* phrase). He says that through human consciousness, our nervous systems can connect with the quantum field and influence the "energy and informational content" of our environment, our world, and our universe, thereby "causing things to manifest in it."

Psychologist and philosopher William James expressed prayer as just such a form of metaphysics: "a process wherein work is really done, and spiritual energy flows in and produces effects, either psychological or material, within the phenomenal world."

Such thoughts are beautiful to contemplate and marvelous to behold, but, somewhat like God himself, their actuality is impossible to substantiate in this world. No one can prove the "Big If." At its gut level, prayer is a plea for help when we need it most. Every person with diabetes on earth can relate to that definition.

A Short Litany of Heartfelt Prayers

So saying, I have tried to make my own regular praying as meaningful as possible to myself and my quest for a better, more fulfilling life.

Over the course of the years since I was diagnosed with diabetes, I have formulated a short litany of prayers that express the sum total of my deepest yearnings as a person with diabetes trying to make the most of my life. It is a blueprint for my greatest needs. It is a wish list of everything I believe is required to live my life to its fullest in the context of diabetes.

My daily prayer, which I repeat in the moments when I am going into meditation, changes from time to time in response to the slings and arrows of outrageous fortune, but in essence, it takes the following form:

- I would like my books to be published.
- I would like my books to be the best I can possibly write.
- I would like my books to benefit many people.
- I would like my writing to support myself, my wife's career, and our lifestyle, humble though it might be.
- I would like my writing to support our deepest aspirations, our causes, our volunteer work, and our travels.

- I would like Martha and me to be of robust health.
- I would like my diabetes to be under control and without diabetic complications, and I would like my oral medication to keep working throughout my life.
- I would like fruitful friendships.
- I would like to continue my running and other exercising with joy and lack of pain.
- I would like peace of mind, happiness, meaning, and satisfaction, through harmony with nature and service to humanity.

Perhaps you feel the same deep-seated urge to pray that I do. Perhaps you feel it out of heartfelt religious conviction, or firm belief in a God you know and trust in your own way. Or perhaps you simply need to find some sense of union in a frightful and alienating universe.

Given the vague nature of my own faith, I will probably never be quite certain why I pray. Perhaps it is because diabetes has inspired me with the knowledge that I need all the help I can get. Or perhaps it is for the reason expressed by some unremembered saint during one of the numerous readings of my Catholic childhood:

"I pray because I must."

A Buddhist with a Dry Martini

Reducing Life to Its Priorities

Most of my friends think I'm putting them on when I observe that the 1950 film version of *Harvey* was one of the most profound movies ever made.

"You mean the one about the big rabbit?"

Yeah, *that* Harvey: the version based on the Pulitzer-Prize-winning play by Mary Chase. It's a film starring Jimmy Stewart as Elwood P. Dowd, a gentle tippler whose best friend and drinking buddy is a six-foot-tall (actually, six-foot-three-and-one-half-inch-tall) Celtic pooka, or faerie-sprite in animal form.

Most people look at the film as a wonderful comedy and farce. I look at *Harvey* as the best role model I've ever found for clarity of ideals and clearness of behavior.

While everyone else in the plot is operating in a frenzy of self-importance, self-seeking, or self-delusion, Elwood regards the world around him with perfect understanding, perfect tolerance, perfect compassion, and perfect acceptance. To me, Elwood P. Dowd is a Buddhist with a dry martini.

"I wrestled for 35 years with reality," Elwood sums up his Zen attitude, "and finally overcame it."

Strange as it sounds to my friends, I have always found great inspiration in this character's unshakable composure, his firm sense of self-identity, and the clearly articulated morality of his behavior. His is an elegant role model, sloshed though he might be, for clarifying one's life into its essential elements. For deciding on one's priorities and living by them.

Just as Elwood P. Dowd was inspired to change and clarify his life by an illusory pooka, I was inspired to clarify mine by my own six-foot-tall rabbit named diabetes.

A Pure Stock of Beliefs

When I use the word "clarify," I think of the way fine cooks clarify a soup stock by introducing egg whites, which rise to the top as the liquid simmers, drawing out all the impurities and leaving the stock clear and ready for use as the basic ingredient in numerous hearty soups.

Likewise, my own clarification is an attempt to clear away the confusion in my life, much as egg whites draw out impurities. It is an attempt to clarify my own ideals into a pure stock of beliefs and change my negative attitudes into positive actions.

As the Dalai Lama once described this process, "The systematic training of the mind means the cultivation of happiness, the genuine inner transformation by deliberately selecting and focusing on positive mental states and challenging negative mental states."

He summed up what I mean by clarification by calling it "positive conditioning."

I have found one mental exercise especially useful for clarifying my priorities and positive conditioning. Over the years since I was diagnosed with diabetes, I have gradually developed a list of basic spiritual principles, something like beatitudes, that I repeat to myself every day. I suppose you might say these beatitudes summarize my whole spiritual philosophy and the means for putting it into action. By repeating them daily, I confirm my resolve to practice what I preach. I also find this exercise a wonderful way to clarify the stock, and take stock in the clarity, of my life.

You might want to create your own set of principles, which express your own priorities, but I will give you my list as a way to begin. In parentheses I also offer a brief explanation of what each of these beatitudes means to me when I say it.

- I will practice truth, compassion, and non-judgment (meaning I will look at life without self-deceit, I will have compassion for all

living things, and will try not to criticize my
fellow human beings).
- I will practice giving and receiving (meaning
  I will try to appreciate all the benefits and
  satisfactions of shared benevolence).
- I will practice self-awareness (meaning I will
  stop for a moment and examine each of my
  emotional reactions to each event that happens
  every day).
- I will practice prayer (meaning I will try to
  connect with the sacred nature of life).
- I will practice acceptance (meaning I will
  totally accept the present as what is meant to
  be, while working to change the future into a
  better time).
- I will practice detachment from my negative
  conditioning (meaning I will attempt to
  distance myself from all the pessimistic
  thinking that has caused me so much grief all
  my life).
- I will practice right conduct (meaning I will
  work to make the world a better place).

Falling Woefully Short

Unfortunately, I don't always live up to my
beatitudes. I often fall woefully short while trying to
reach the ambitious goals they set. But at least these
beliefs let me know exactly what I am trying to do with
my life on a daily basis. If one has nothing to live up to,
one will have plenty to live down.

One more way I have tried to practice clarification is by making the mechanics of my life conform to my newfound ideals.

As you have seen in the autobiographical sections of this book, diabetes made me realize that I needed a big attitude adjustment. Every person with diabetes does. One of my most important decisions after being diagnosed with diabetes was to make the overall body of my writing worthwhile, constructive, and socially meaningful.

In Eastern philosophies, such a decision is part of practicing dharma, which entails making a conscious effort to "do the right thing" all the time in conjunction with the natural moral laws of the universe. It was for this reason that I quit my rather meaningless job at UMass, set out on a spiritual pilgrimage, and attempted to write material that would have a positive impact on the people who read it.

Making Peace with Myself

I have found that it is critical for me, as a person with diabetes, to feel that what I am doing with my life makes a difference in the world around me. I can most easily make such a difference by using my most useful gift and talent, my writing.

For other people with diabetes, their gifts and talents will be of a different kind. Each must find his or her own approach to dharma. Each must find his or her own unique form of right conduct.

I realize that every job cannot be terribly meaningful, and that every person with diabetes might not be in a financial or social position to seek alternative employment. However, your daily routine can be spiritually augmented in many ways.

Perhaps the most righteous employment of all, and certainly the most difficult, is raising a loving family and giving your children healthy values. As one Peace Corps slogan goes, "It's the hardest job you'll ever love." Unfortunately, it's also a job that many of us, including myself, have either avoided or failed to carry out in a responsible manner.

Another way to find meaning is by volunteering your spare time in worthy causes. To list just a few kinds of volunteer work, these jobs might include:

- being a big brother or big sister
- offering your services to the Red Cross
- taking part in the socially responsible activities run by so many churches, synagogues, fraternal organizations, and clubs
- volunteering to work for a political candidate whose policies you believe in
- working for your local Audubon sanctuary or state park
- distributing Meals on Wheels
- taking pledge calls for your public radio or television station
- providing recreation activities for a local cerebral palsy support group
- serving at your local Special Olympics

The opportunities are endless for those who want to do public service. If time and family commitments keep you from doing volunteer activities, you can support a foreign foster child, or donate to worthy environmental organizations, or subscribe to an activist network devoted to contacting Congressional representatives. Do anything that makes you feel like you're making a difference by living up to your values and beliefs.

One of the best examples of social action I know is a Cambodian monk named Maha Goshananda, who has spent much of his life removing unexploded land mines left behind a quarter-century ago by the Khmer Rouge. When he was once asked to explain why he did such difficult and dangerous work, his answer summarized the reasoning behind right conduct for everyone.

"I am making peace with myself."

This Is What You Shall Do

More than 150 years ago, the wondrous poet Walt Whitman set down the best possible formula for right action, and I don't believe anyone has improved upon it since then.

"This is what you shall do: Love the earth and sun and the animals, despise riches, give alms to everyone that asks, stand up for the stupid and crazy, devote your income and labor to others, hate tyrants, argue not concerning God, have patience and indulgence toward the people, re-examine all you have been told at school or church or in any book, dismiss what insults your very soul, and your very flesh shall become a poem."

If you can do all *that*, you can join the ranks of Mahatma Gandhi, Albert Schweitzer, Helen Keller, Black Elk, Martin Luther King, Jr., Rachel Carson, Cesar Chavez, Mother Theresa, and the Dalai Lama as the saints and holy people of our times.

If so, you can also throw away this book. You don't need my advice about right conduct or anything else.

Afterthought

A Few Last Words About the
Pursuit of Mystery

At the risk of branding myself as the oddball I probably am, I must add a final note about one more spiritual practice that I've found makes life much more worthwhile and exhilarating. I call it "the pursuit of mystery." By that I mean an active quest for all those phenomena that to me symbolize the rich, cosmic, and fathomless essence of life. One afternoon, during my daily exercise routine, I found myself in the center of Crystal Lake as I rested from a strenuous stint of swimming by paddling languidly on the surface. As I floated there, belly-up and facing the sky, I suddenly felt as though I were stretched between two facing mirrors, reflecting the infinite secrets of the universe. I sensed I could slip through a glass darkly in either direction.

I mused in this position for some moments, as the water rippled against my skin like a soft chant, and soon realized that no person alive or dead—no Einstein, no Sagan, no Hawkins, no Aristotle, no Galileo—could comprehend even a small percentage of what makes up reality in the surrounding cosmos.

If I rose through the looking glass in one direction, nobody could ever explain the astronomical forces that make the immense galaxies work. Likewise, if I sank through the looking glass in the other direction, nobody could ever totally fathom the minute chemical reactions, biological processes, and energy exchanges that make even so small a world as a pond function.

In other words, we're all living in Wonderland.

A Society of Debunkers

In our state of know-nothingness, though, we have the arrogance to mock and ridicule and scoff at all those mysteries we can neither observe with our senses, measure with our instruments, nor conceive with our imaginations. At the same time as our science derides religion for condemning any scientific evidence that doesn't fit into a sacrosanct paradigm, we have turned science into a religion itself, which condemns any mysterious evidence that doesn't fit into its own sacrosanct paradigm.

Thus we have become a society of debunkers whose reaction to people who explore the inexplicable is to label them as nutcases.

And what a lot we are missing in our close-mindedness. I am not at all sure whether I believe in such marvels as UFOs, ghosts, Bigfoot, time travel, alien abductions, crop circles, astrology, witch's spells, remote viewing, beatific visions, reincarnation, astro-travel, and the Loch Ness Monster. But what a boring existence this would be without them. What a limiting mindset to be locked into a purely material world, with truly materialistic ideals, and a solely materialistic reality. What a drag to have all the answers and none of the questions.

By contrast, what an invigorating experience it is to open one's mind to the totality of experience floating like an atomic shadow beyond the limits of the "real" world.

Slip into the Night Stream

My friend Al Hall terms the far-side of reality as the "Night Stream." It can be found coursing through the wee hours of the morning on talk shows peopled variously by insomniacs, paranoids, truth seekers, hard-core believers, fanatics, madmen, and those inquisitive souls gently obsessed with the otherworldly manifestations that give life its depth perception.

My own attitude is that I prefer to accept the possibility of all these mysteries, simply because they make life much more fascinating. Since I was diagnosed with diabetes, I have begun delving into all the bewitching uncertainties of life as it evolves, mutates, and blossoms, and I have never been happier.

I know this exploration of mine makes me seem an odd duck to my less mystical associates. For example, Martha and I recently hosted a young house guest who prided himself on his scientific attitude, and during our evening conversation I found myself expressing some of my more unorthodox views about the possible consequences of global warming, the concept of spirits as time travelers, and the intentions of the alien beings behind the UFO phenomenon.

By the hard glint in our young friend's pupils and the skeptical look on his face, I could tell he was lumping me with all the other screwballs he had encountered throughout his life.

It became clear to me during this conversation that somehow in the past few years since I was diagnosed with diabetes, and without me ever being aware of it, I had passed through whatever invisible barrier separates the angry young man I used to be from the eccentric old kook I am now. I had entered the lunatic fringe.

With that initiation, then, I invite you to try kookhood yourself. It is one of the many fringe benefits that come with membership in the community of people with diabetes everywhere. I sometimes look at diabetes as a license to explore all the wonders that protocol, inhibitions, and good form prohibited in the past. By learning to live every day as though it were my last, as diabetes has taught me, I have become much more daring and resourceful in the eccentricities I am willing to entertain.

Diabetes has served as my passport to the uncanny. Go ahead, my friend. As one last spiritual experiment, take the plunge yourself. Slip into the Night Stream.

Outer Most Radio

I recently finished writing an article about community radio station WOMR (which stands for "Outer Most Radio") in Provincetown, at the tip of Cape Cod. This station is a sort of Twilight Zone of the airwaves whose station manager once summarized the programming as "strangely beautiful and beautifully strange."

My wife Martha and I have developed a little routine during our ten years of listening to this zany station and its bizarre broadcasting. Every time something odd and wonderful would play on WOMR, we would turn to each other and simultaneously mouth the words "Outer Most Radio."

Later, our routine evolved into a way to express anything anywhere with an "outer most" quality to it. "Outer Most Radio," we found ourselves repeating as the sweet mystery of life revealed itself in its many facets.

"Splendiferous!" is the way Zorba the Greek expressed this same kind of phenomenon.

To me "Outer Most Radio" has become a kind of mantra, not unlike the way author Kurt Vonnegut used "So it goes" as a refrain to express the whimsical and unexplainable nature of life in his novel *Slaughterhouse-five*.

My final piece of spiritual advice for you is to go forth and explore all the rich texture life has to offer.

Hobnob with the splendiferous. Rub elbows with the lunatic fringe. And when you come across one of those exquisite mysteries that should make us all feel at once humbled and ecstatic, then repeat after me:

"Outer Most Radio."

"Outer Most Radio."

"Outer Most Radio."

"Outer Most Radio."

- END -

Charles Creekmore has been a professional journalist since 1974, and a person with diabetes since 1996. His writing has been featured in numerous periodicals, including *Psychology Today, Omni, Modern Maturity, Islands, National Wildlife, Runner's World, Travel & Leisure*, the *Utne Reader*, the *Boston Globe, USA Today*, and the *New York Times Syndicate*. He is also a poet whose verse has appeared in *Prism International, The Fiddlehead, The Malcontent, Wascana Review, Asylum, Queens Quarterly, Bouillabaisse, Howling Dog*, and other literary journals. A graduate of the University of Massachusetts-Amherst, he has served variously as a VISTA, Peace Corps, and United Nations volunteer, and a member of a biological expedition tracking monarch butterflies to their wintering sites in the mountains of central Mexico. He lives on Cape Cod in Massachusetts.

Index

Best-sellers from the
American Diabetes Association

American Diabetes Association
Complete Guide to Diabetes, Second edition
Everything you ever needed to know about diabetes in one practical book. It covers everything from how to manage types 1, 2, and gestational diabetes, to traveling with insulin, sick-day action plans, and recognizing hypoglycemia, as well as:
• Symptoms • Complications • Exercise and nutrition
• Blood sugar control • Sexual issues • Drug therapies
• Insulin regimes • More
458 pages, softcover.
#4809-02 Nonmember: $23.95 Member: $19.95

101 Tips for Simplifying Diabetes
American Diabetes Association
An exciting new edition to the best selling ADA 101 tips series. Open it up to find all kinds of helpful, practical ammunition to get—and keep—the upper hand when dealing with diabetes. If nighttime blood sugar lows concern you, learn how an alarm clock can help you simplify this problem. If finger pricks cause you pain just thinking about them, try the "milking your finger" trick—it works. You might even outsmart heart disease. Ask your doctor about this new drug—it could just be your "ace" in the hole. Plus, look at all of these other terrific ways to get the upper hand:

• Simplify your diabetes care—try this new insulin that only needs to be taken once a day.
• Conquer cravings that sabotage your diet—eat this yummy berry to ward off hunger fast.
• Prevent holiday weight gain—retrain your brain to reach for this delicious dessert instead of fat-packed pie.

Blood sugar, medications, meal plans, exercise, nutrition—it's all in this new 101 tips book that shows you how to outsmart diabetes. 128 pages, softcover
#4847-01 One low price: $14.95

When Diabetes Hits Home
Wendy Satin Rapaport, LCSW, PsyD
Effective strategies for coping with the ups and downs of diabetes. Throughout your life you and those you love will experience a range of emotions as the trials and tribulations of diabetes come and go. Here and now get effective strategies for coping. 289 pages, softcover.
#4818-01 Nonmember: $19.95 Member: $17.95

The "I Hate to Exercise" Book for People with Diabetes
Charlotte Hayes, MMSc, MS, RD, CDE
Bid vigorous exercise goodbye. All you need is 30 minutes a day and our new plan to get all the benefits without all the sweat. You'll be amazed at how a simple everyday activity like walking, cutting the grass, or watching TV can become an opportunity to strengthen your heart and muscles, improve your diabetes control, and more. Get all the insight you need to get started—even if you've never exercised before—and create goals and stick to them. 128 pages, softcover.
#4837-01 Nonmember: $14.95 Member: $12.95

Diabetes Meal Planning Made Easy, Second edition
Hope Warsaw, MMSc, RD, CDE
The diabetes food pyramid doesn't have to be complicated—even if you live life in the fast lane. In fact, it's downright easy to follow—and can help you simplify your life. Learn how to:

- Easily eat more fruits and vegetables
- Skim off nasty fat grams
- Eat like a champion away from home

Get the latest nutrition recommendations, the low down on vitamins and minerals, and the real truth behind health claims made
on food labels. 235 pages, softcover.
#4706-02 Nonmember: $14.95 Member: $12.95

Type 2 Diabetes:
Your Healthy Living Guide, Third edition
American Diabetes Association
Tips, techniques, and practical advice to keep you in charge of
your life. By understanding how and when to check your blood
sugar and what to do with the results, you can free yourself from
complications that can interfere with your daily living. Know
which signs signal "do something quick" and get expert advice
on what to do. Here are recent updates on medications and monitoring. Find sage advice for handling diabetes in the workplace.
More. 176 pages, softcover.
#4804-03 Nonmember: $16.95 Member: $14.95

Caring for the Diabetic Soul
American Diabetes Association
Success strategies for coping with the emotional stress of diabetes. Get a new outlook on life. Maintain emotional balance.
Face your feelings and confront your fears. Realize your dreams
and rebuild your hope. An easy, fast read, this popular book
helps you cope with denial, control stress and anger, build self-
esteem, give perfection the big push off, and use humor to defuse
potentially explosive situations.
213 pages, softcover.
#4815-01 Nonmember: $9.95 Member: $8.95

Diabetes Burnout:
What to Do When You Can't Take It Anymore
William H. Polonsky, PhD, CDE
Banish burnout and depression. Living with diabetes is hard. It's
easy to get discouraged, frustrated, and burned out. Here's an
author that understands the emotional rollercoaster and gives

you the tools you need to keep from being overwhelmed. Written with compassion and a sprinkle of humor. 350 pages, softcover.
#4822-01 Nonmember: $18.95 Member: $16.95

Meditations on Diabetes
Catherine Feste, MA
Ancient and modern wise "men" and healers reveal secrets to improving your diabetes. Gain an inner peace and calming strength. Draw on the healing wisdom of people like Ralph Waldo Emerson, Eleanor Roosevelt, Helen Keller, and others. 264 pages, softcover.
#4820-01 Nonmember: $13.95 Member: $11.95

About the American Diabetes Association

The American Diabetes Association is the nation's leading voluntary health organization supporting diabetes research, information, and advocacy. Its mission is to prevent and cure diabetes and to improve the lives of all people affected by diabetes. The American Diabetes Association is the leading publisher of comprehensive diabetes information. Its huge library of practical and authoritative books for people with diabetes covers every aspect of self-care—cooking and nutrition, fitness, weight control, medications, complications, emotional issues, and general self-care.

To order American Diabetes Association books: Call 1-800-232-6733. http://store.diabetes.org [Note: there is no need to use **www** when typing this particular Web address]

To join the American Diabetes Association: Call 1-800-806-7801. www.diabetes.org/membership

For more information about diabetes or ADA programs and services: Call 1-800-342-2383. E-mail: Customerservice@diabetes.org www.diabetes.org

To locate an ADA/NCQA Recognized Provider of quality diabetes care in your area: Call 1-703-549-1500 ext. 2202. www.diabetes.org/recognition/Physicians/ListAll.asp

To find an ADA Recognized Education Program in your area: Call 1-888-232-0822. www.diabetes.org/recognition/education.asp

To join the fight to increase funding for diabetes research, end discrimination, and improve insurance coverage: Call 1-800-342-2383. www.diabetes.org/advocacy

To find out how you can get involved with the programs in your community: Call 1-800-342-2383. See below for program Web addresses.

- *American Diabetes Month:* Educational activities aimed at those diagnosed with diabetes—month of November. www.diabetes.org/ADM
- *American Diabetes Alert:* Annual public awareness campaign to find the undiagnosed—held the fourth Tuesday in March. www.diabetes.org/alert
- *The Diabetes Assistance & Resources Program (DAR):* diabetes awareness program targeted to the Latino community. www.diabetes.org/DAR
- *African American Program:* diabetes awareness program targeted to the African American community. www.diabetes.org/africanamerican
- *Awakening the Spirit: Pathways to Diabetes Prevention & Control:* diabetes awareness program targeted to the Native American community. www.diabetes.org/awakening

To find out about an important research project regarding type 2 diabetes: www.diabetes.org/ada/research.asp

To obtain information on making a planned gift or charitable bequest: Call 1-888-700-7029. www.diabetes.org/ada/plan.asp

To make a donation or memorial contribution: Call 1-800-342-2383. www.diabetes.org/ada/cont.asp